Long-Term Pain

A guide to practical management

Edited by

John Lee

Consultant in Pain Medicine, Honorary Senior Lecturer and Lead Clinician at the Pain Management Centre, University College London Hospitals, the National Hospital for Neurology and Neurosurgery, Queen Square, London, UK

and

Andrew Baranowski

Consultant in Pain Medicine and Honorary Senior Lecturer at the Pain Management Centre, University College London Hospitals, the National Hospital for Neurology and Neurosurgery, Queen Square, London, UK

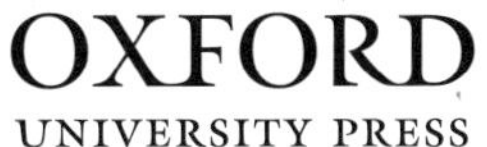
OXFORD UNIVERSITY PRESS

OXFORD
UNIVERSITY PRESS

Great Clarendon Street, Oxford OX2 6DP

Oxford University Press is a department of the University of Oxford.
It furthers the University's objective of excellence in research, scholarship,
and education by publishing worldwide in

Oxford New York

Auckland Cape Town Dar es Salaam Hong Kong Karachi
Kuala Lumpur Madrid Melbourne Mexico City Nairobi
New Delhi Shanghai Taipei Toronto

With offices in

Argentina Austria Brazil Chile Czech Republic France Greece
Guatemala Hungary Italy Japan Poland Portugal Singapore
South Korea Switzerland Thailand Turkey Ukraine Vietnam

Published in the United States
by Oxford University Press, Inc., New York

First published 2007

British Library Cataloguing in Publication Data
Data available

Library of Congress Cataloging in Publication Data
Data available

Typeset by Newgen Imaging Systems (P) Ltd., Chennai, India
Printed in Italy
on acid-free paper by
Legoprint S.p.A.

ISBN 0–19–921415–8 978–0–19–921415–0

10 9 8 7 6 5 4 3 2 1

Contents

Contributors

Andrew Baranowski
Consultant in Pain Medicine, University College London Hospitals, UK
Chapter 11 Pain of urological and genital origin

Brigitta Brandner
Consultant Anaesthetist with an interest in Pain, University College London Hospitals, UK
Chapter 4 Some treatments cause chronic pain: can we reduce the risk?

Lesley Bromley
Senior Lecturer in Anaesthesia, University College London, UK
Chapter 2 Mechanisms of acute pain

Sam Chong
Consultant Neurologist, King's College Hospital, London, UK
Chapter 9 Prescribing for people with pain originating in the nervous system. Part 2 Anticonvulsants

James de Courcy
Consultant in Pain Management with an interest in Palliative Care, Cheltenham General Hospital, UK
Chapter 12 Cancer pain

Simon Davies
Consultant Anaesthetist with an interest in Pain, Great Western Hospital, Swindon, UK
Chapter 8 Prescribing for people with pain originating in the nervous system. Part 1 Tricyclic anti-depressants

Simon Dolin
Consultant in Pain Medicine, St Richard's Hospital, Chichester, UK
Chapter 7 What should I feel like after treatment at the pain clinic?

Jon Francis
Consultant in Pain Medicine, Cheltenham General Hospital, UK
Chapter 10 Strong opioids in the treatment of people with non-malignant pain

Sian Jaggar
Consultant Anaesthetist with an interest in Pain, Royal Brompton National Heart and Lung Hospital, London, UK
Chapter 1 Why do some pains become chronic?

John Lee
Consultant in Pain Medicine, University College London Hospitals, UK
Chapter 6 Injections, invasive treatments and the 'whole patient' view

Anna Mandeville
Consultant Clinical Psychologist, University College London Hospitals, UK
Chapter 13 Psychological aspects of pain

Mary Newton
Consultant Neuroanaesthetist, National Hospital for Neurology and Neurosurgery, London, UK
Chapter 3 Pharmacological targets in acute pain

Cathy Price
Consultant in Pain Medicine, Southampton General Hospital, UK
Chapter 16 Getting back to work

Kate Ridout
Consultant Clinical Psychologist, University College London Hospitals, UK
Chapter 13 Psychological aspects of pain

Andrew Souter
Consultant in Pain Medicine, Royal United Hospital, Bath, UK
Chapter 5 Assessing people with longstanding pain

Trudy Towell
Nurse Consultant, Queen's Medical Centre, Nottingham, UK
Chapter 15 Working across boundaries in pain medicine

Lucy Ward
Consultant in Pain Medicine, Royal Free Hospital, London, UK
Chapter 7 What should I feel like after treatment at the pain clinic?

Kelly Wynne
IME Quality Assurance Programme Co-ordinator, Victorian Workcover Authority, Melbourne, Australia
Chapter 14 Non-medical treatment in managing people with long-term pain

Preface

This is a pocket book about patients who suffer long-term pain. It is designed for primary care clinicians (for example doctors, nurses, physiotherapists, occupational therapists or pharmacists) who want to learn more about the treatment of people with long-term pain. It is written in a distinct style to take the development of ideas about pain from the simple to the complex during the course of a chapter, and the course of the book. The information provided is up to date and relevant for the treatment of patients in long term pain written by doctors who's practise is either wholly or substantially related to people with pain. It is not intended to be an exhaustive text; it provides relevant examples of everyday patients with their problems to provide carers with the confidence to prescribe and treat patients with more difficult pain. A starting list of references is given, where appropriate, and links to internet resources have also been provided.

The book emphasizes the need to consider the triumvirate of biological, psychological and social impacts of pain. Details of the science behind common conditions and their remedies are also given in a chatty style in an attempt to demystify areas of medicine that are often seen as problematic. The book is extensively edited to provide the consistent style; most chapters use actual cases around which the theme of the chapter is developed to maintain the 'hands-on' nature of the text.

Chapter 1

Why do some pains become chronic?

Sian Jaggar

Chronic pain happens for many different reasons and not only as a consequence of tissue injury. There are also many different risk factors. This chapter describes two patients and how pain becomes long term for the second.

1.1 Andrew has back pain

Andrew is a 58-year-old university lecturer. He was lifting a pile of papers in his office two days ago when 'something suddenly went'. He has already been taking paracetamol and ibuprofen regularly and has now come to see his GP as he is irritated by his pain and the disability it is causing. Andrew has been continuing to work during this episode. However, he is concerned to make sure he does not damage himself further. He is normally an active man and his favourite hobby is rambling. He has had to reduce the amount of exercise he does because of his pain.

There is nothing remarkable to find when he is examined. He has a full range of movement with mild discomfort on forward flexion. There is some mild tenderness over the paraspinal muscles in the lumbar region, but no evidence of motor or sensory abnormalities in the lower limbs.

Andrew's GP explains that damage to important tissues or nerves is unlikely to have occurred. He is encouraged to continue light exercises and to gradually increase what he does to work up to a resumption of his normal rambling. She also advises that it may be necessary to take the drugs he is on for a few weeks to help through his period of pain and ensure that he does not lose mobility or strength. Andrew's GP points out that exercise, far from being harmful, is likely to help his recovery and health in the long term.

Andrew is given some leaflets about back care that are available in the surgery. There is a section on general back care with reference to bending and lifting which is pointed out to him to help prevent future incidents. His GP also tells him to come back if the pain is still difficult to control in four weeks time, or if he suffers any shooting pains, numbness in his legs or difficulty passing urine.

Six months later Andrew returns to see his local doctor to obtain a prescription for antimalarial tablets as he is off on a trip to climb Kilimanjaro. He reports to her that his back pain resolved three weeks after it began and has not returned.

This case illustrates the importance of reassurance and continued graded exercise and activity. Bed rest and avoiding activity are well proven to be detrimental to long-term outcomes in people with simple acute back injuries. This GP has reduced Andrew's anxieties about his condition and explained that he has not sustained any serious damage.

Simple musculoskeletal pains can often be best treated

- with a short period of rest followed by
- reassurance alongside
- continued monitored graded exercise and activity

1.2 Alison has breast cancer

Alison is 28-years-old and found a lump in her left breast four months ago. She was seen by her local doctor who immediately sent her to the oncology clinic. Within a month a lumpectomy had been performed. Unexpectedly, this proved to be malignant and she returned for wide local excision with axillary clearance soon after. She felt much relieved when all the nodes were reported clear of tumour and underwent a four week course of radiotherapy. She now has a severe 'dragging' pain in her left axilla and has gone to see her GP.

When Alison's GP takes a careful history, it seems that this dragging pain has been present since the time of her surgery. In the early stages of her recovery she suffered severe postoperative pain and felt that the hospital doctors were not taking her complaints seriously. The day after her operation, the pain was the 'worst I have ever experienced'. Alison then had intermittent morphine injections that relieved her pain but produced severe nausea. Since discharge, she has used a combination of paracetamol and ibuprofen but her pain deteriorated when she started radiotherapy. She now feels unable to return to her job as a secretary at the local school. She feels that being left-handed she would not be able to perform effectively with an arm she didn't want to 'stress and further damage'.

These are not the only things troubling Alison, who is quite tearful during the interview. She thinks her husband is concerned that she is not doing so much around the house. His job is extremely demanding

Non-surgical trauma can cause iatrogenic tissue damage

- radiotherapy
- chemotherapy

In malignant disease, new pain is often due to recurrence of tumour.

at the moment and she feels that he is expecting her to do more than she can. Memories of her childhood have been troubling Alison; she remembers that her father died suddenly whilst painting the kitchen.

Andrew's back pain in the first case history seemed straightforward. For Alison it is clear that her pain is multifactorial where multimodal therapeutic targets may all help (i.e. drugs, physical therapies, psychological support and the provision of physical aids).

Features which may increase the likelihood of long-term pain and disability

- a history of severe pain
- a family history of susceptibility to pain
- worry that pain may be due to a disease that reduces life expectancy
- depression and anxiety
- fear of injury
- secondary gains (e.g. a higher income on benefits than when at work)
- inappropriate family support:
  - too little, which encourages increasing complaints in an attempt to gain sympathy
  - too much, which encourages withdrawal and dependence
- pending litigation
- low social class
- lower levels of income

Alison continues to visit her GP every month. She is hoping for a drug that will 'cure' her pain. She requires a great deal of support. At one point her GP suggests counselling for Alison and her husband, which they decline. She would like to have children, but feels that she will not be able to cope with being a working mother. Over the next few years Alison remains resistant to the idea that psychological support may help her. She is happy to try new drugs and physical therapies (including acupuncture and transcutaneous electrical nerve stimulation (TENS)) but is quite clear that her pain is 'not in her head'. Her cancer does not recur.

1.3 Summary

For Alison, a combination of surgery and radiotherapy has left her with pain that is poorly responsive to medication and physical measures. She also has a number of other concerns that she seems unable to tackle effectively herself. Treatment that will give her psychosocial support may be the most effective therapy: it needs to recognize all the different parts that make up who she is, including her important relationships, aspirations and work environment. Despite clinicians' best intentions, many patients will not accept the treatment that is appropriate and support can only be provided in a format that is comfortable, such as a GP's surgery.

Chapter 2

Mechanisms of acute pain

Lesley Bromley

Our increasing understanding of how the nervous system detects painful stimuli, and how it deals with the information has improved acute pain management. Since prehistory it has been evident that the nervous system conducted information to the brain. Philosophers such as Descartes thought the nerves 'opened up pores in the common sense centre'. We know that the old idea of the nerves as a form of wiring is too simplistic and that the nervous system is able to modify the information that arrives at every synapse along the way to the brain. This chapter explains the current science behind the development of pain when tissue damage first occurs.

2.1 Ron has an inguinal herniorraphy

Ron Evans is 65-years-old, he had a hernia repaired as a day case and has been at home 24 h. He is anxious because he has quite a lot of pain from the site of the operation and around the area of the wound. The pain is much worse if he moves about.

Ron's experience provides an opportunity to examine the mechanisms of acute pain. The surgeon who repaired his hernia produced tissue damage in the superficial and deeper layers of his abdominal wall. This released cell contents into the wound. These chemicals triggered cascades that produce transmitters stimulating the primary afferent sensory nerves lying in the tissues.

The term 'sensitizing soup' has been used to describe this solution of chemicals. The best known cascade is the prostaglandin system, but bradykinins, purines such as adenosine triphosphate, and ions such as potassium and hydrogen, can stimulate receptors in sensory nerves.

Other chemicals affect the sensitivity of nerves include:

- nerve growth factor (NGF), which upregulates bradykinin binding
- capsaicin (the 'heat' in chillies) which acts on the vanilloid receptor (normally sensitive to H^+ ions)
- cannabinoid receptors that seem to be related to the bradykinin/NGF system.

Transmitters known to stimulate primary sensory nerves
• prostaglandins
• histamine
• adenosine triphosphate (ATP)
• potassium ions (K^+)
• hydrogen ions (H^+)
• bradykinins
• 5-hydroxytryptamine (5-HT, serotonin)
• substance P

New analgesic drugs will come from a better understanding of the relationships between the chemicals released from nerves, the reflex responses they initiate, and the interactions with other systems such as the mediators from white blood cells. For Ron, non-steroidal anti-inflammatory drugs (NSAIDs) disrupt the prostaglandin pathway and he would benefit from starting an NSAID and with the addition of regular paracetamol.

It is interesting to go through the different steps in the transmission of 'pain' as it is not only a fascinating tale, but also clarifies why so many different types of drugs can modulate sensations from the world around us. The first step is to appreciate that pain is the end result, the sense perceived by the individual. The correct term for the process that results in pain is nociception, which requires an intact central nervous system. The nociceptive pathways may be activated without pain being perceived such as in a decerebrate animal. Information from the area of the wound in Ron's groin travels in the primary nociceptive sensory nerves entering the dorsal horn of the spinal cord. In the dorsal horn the primary nerves relay with the secondary afferent nerves. This is the site of Melzac and Wall's 'gate'. Nociceptive primary sensory nerves are of two types according to size. The Aδ-fibres are thinly myelinated, medium-sized in diameter and conduct pain quickly, the 'ouch' type of pain. They synapse in laminas I and V of the dorsal horn. C-Fibres are unmyelinated, smaller and synapse in lamina I; they conduct more slowly and transmit dull, aching pain.

Information arriving at the dorsal horn is modified before it passes in the lateral spinothalamic tracts to the brain. It can be amplified before travelling onwards, known as 'central sensitization', or 'suppressed', for instance by the interaction of descending pathways. The nerves coming into the spinal cord transmitting messengers release neurotransmitters; glutamate is the major constituent, but other substances (neurokinins and substance P, both neuromodulators) are also present. The neuromodulators alter the sensitivity of the neurons. The synapses have many different receptors both pre- and postsynaptically which are all targets for drugs to reduce pain. These receptors include those for opioids, 5-HT, adenosine, glycine, gamma-amino butyric acid (GABA), neurokinin-1 and α_2-adrenoreceptors.

Central sensitization amplifies the signals occurring in the deep layer, lamina V. Incoming action potentials reach a certain electrical threshold that opens NMDA receptors, producing many more firings in the secondary nerve. The brain interprets this as increasing pain.

Descending pathways can suppress the signal. These pathways include the α_2-adrenoreceptors that are also stimulated by circulating adrenaline and noradrenaline. This is part of the explanation of 'battlefield analgesia' where soldiers feel no pain from serious wounds while in the battle and only feel the pain later in the safety of field hospital. Their circulating adrenaline is so high in battle that pain is 'turned off' for the duration. When his daughter rings the door bell, Ron may notice that his pain is less noticeable; adrenaline released in response to the surprise of the sound and the anticipation of seeing his daughter suppresses the pain.

The third effect bought about in the dorsal horn is that of receptive field enlargement. Ron complains of pain and aching in the area around the wound. The tissue is intact, there is no peripheral sensitizing soup, yet there is pain. This extended pain is caused by changes in the threshold of the nerves in the dorsal horn surrounding those that have received input from the damaged tissue. The receptive field is enlarged around the damaged area and the nerves are more easily stimulated. Sensations that are not normally painful may start to feel painful, for example light touch, and Ron feels pain when the area around the dressing is touched some distance from his wound. This is called allodynia. Opioids such as dihydrocodeine or tramadol (which has actions at both opioid receptors and α_2-adrenoreceptors) are useful analgesics here. Ron might take one of these before the dressing is changed.

Pain phenomena from the dorsal horn

1. Central sensitization—mechanisms for increasing the signal
2. Hyperaesthesia—increased receptive field, where the perception of non-painful signals is increased
3. Secondary hyperalgesia—increased receptive field, where the perception of painful signals is increased
4. Allodynia—pain due to a stimulus that does not normally provoke pain

Travelling up to the brain, the nerves pass through the brain stem which is rich in opioid receptors and is another site of drug action. This is very close to the respiratory centre and is involved in the mechanism of respiratory depression seen with opioids. The nerves then pass through the thalamus which is a further site of modification of the signal and about which very little is known. Finally the information is projected to the cortex where the nociceptive signal is perceived as pain. The thalamus and cortex have interactions with the limbic system, with the memory and the emotions. After leaving hospital, Ron may feel anxious and insecure at first when returning home, making pain seem worse.

Science has begun to understand all of the events that Ron experiences. He can be reassured that his pain will reduce in intensity as healing takes place and that acute pain of this type should be short lived and self-limiting. Some of the themes and the mechanisms that we have discussed in this chapter about acute pain are pertinent in the development of long-term pain so it is useful to talk about them at this early stage.

2.2 Jenny's sprained ankle

Jenny is a 15-year-old schoolgirl. She fell over on the netball court and hurt her ankle. She can walk on the ankle, but it is swollen and painful despite no bruising. Jenny has suffered acute trauma without surgical tissue disruption. The sprained ankle will have some tearing of soft-tissue structures and the same mechanism will apply to generating pain as in Ron's hernia operation. The whole ankle will be painful with significant central sensitization. Allodynia may also be a feature. Jenny's anxiety that she may not be able to play in her next netball match may increase her perception of pain. She can be reassured that her pain will resolve over a number of weeks as her ankle heals, the spinal cord receives less input from the periphery and the enlarged receptive fields return to their normal representation in the dorsal horn.

2.3 Summary

- Acute pain from tissue damage is usually self-limiting.
- Nociceptive impulses are generated in primary sensory nerves by chemical mediators released around damaged tissues.
- The spinal cord receives these impulses in the dorsal horn where they can be amplified by repetitive stimulation, or reduced by peripheral input such as by means of a transcutaneous nerve stimulator or as a result of activating descending pathways.

- In the spinal cord the representation of the painful area and the sensitivity of other surrounding areas can be modified.
- Modification can also take place at the level of the brain stem and thalamus.
- The perception of the pain is altered by higher emotions such as anxiety and fear.

Chapter 3

Pharmacological targets in acute pain

Mary Newton

This chapter employs some of the targets that were discussed in the last chapter. It describes the management of two patients with severe acute pain. The first one has acute musculoskeletal pain, and the second, a combination of musculoskeletal and neuropathic pain. The chapter emphasizes the importance of regular analgesia, co-analgesia and non-pharmacological adjuncts.

3.1 Rosie fractured her humerus

Rosie is 62-years-old. She broke the neck of her left humerus three weeks ago when she slipped on ice. This was managed conservatively with a collar and cuff. Initially she had severe pain in her arm but this has almost completely resolved and now she needs only the occasional paracetamol in the evening.

Rosie is a highly motivated lady and was looking forward to mobilizing her arm so that she could help with looking after her young grandchildren again. When the collar and cuff came off, she had excruciating pain in her shoulder and she was unable to comply with the simple exercises that she had been given to perform. She naturally thought that something had been overlooked and that something was seriously the matter with her arm.

Rosie sought an urgent appointment with her GP. Examination revealed a shoulder which was tender around the coracoid process. Active and passive movements were restricted by pain. She rated her pain as 2/10 at rest and 8/10 on movement. Rosie's doctor explained that she almost certainly had a frozen shoulder and she was greatly relieved to have an explanation of her pain which she could understand.

It was explained that a frozen shoulder is fairly common following fractures of this type and that, despite the pain, it was essential that she continued with her programme of gentle shoulder movements. Her GP prescribed regular paracetamol and ibuprofen for two weeks. Rosie was encouraged to place a warm or cold pack over her shoulder before movement to see if either brought relief.

This combination of therapy helped but Rosie still reported pain scores of 6/10 on exercise. Her GP recommended that Rosie should take codeine phosphate regularly in addition to the other medications to facilitate exercise and gave her a further two week supply. With this combination her pain scores fell to 3/10 during her exercises. She was referred to the local physiotherapy department six weeks after her fracture when bony fusion would allow antigravity exercises. The 'step-up' in activity again was very painful and Rosie took paracetamol before each treatment session. Nine months after her initial injury she had regained almost a complete range of movement in the affected shoulder.

3.2 Katie's back pain

Katie, a 33-year-old housewife, requested a home visit from her GP for severe back pain which had resulted in immobility. The only problem she had seen her GP for in the past was a duodenal ulcer three years ago (confirmed by endoscopy). This had resolved following a course of a proton pump inhibitor.

Lying on her bed, she recounted how after months of grumbling low back pain she had awoken that morning with excruciating pain in the same area. Katie described the pain as a severe ache in her lower back. There was no radiation of the pain but it was exacerbated by movement, especially bending forward. Katie had taken two separate doses of paracetamol but this had very little effect. On examination, Katie was clearly in severe discomfort. She had muscle spasm in her lumbar region and could not tolerate any straight leg raising. Pain scores were explained and Katie rated her pain as 8/10 at rest and 10/10 on movement.

During the consultation Katie volunteered that she had nursed her mother dying from carcinoma of the breast with multiple bony metastases and was terrified that her own pain was due to 'bone cancer'. She was enormously reassured to learn that she almost certainly had severe muscle spasm possibly secondary to damage to a lumbar intervertebral disc. The problem was common and well understood. The anatomy of the lumbar spine and intervertebral discs was explained in simple terms. Katie was told that the leaked contents of the ruptured disc were highly irritant (containing high concentrations of prostaglandins) and had caused inflammation in the surrounding tissues. She was told that about 70% of cases improved in a week or two and resolved completely with conservative measures in a few months' time.

Pain relief is often improved by

- explanation
- appropriate reassurance
- regular analgesia
- co-analgesia
- gentle mobilization

Titration of analgesia can be usefully guided by:

- pain scores—visual analogue or verbal rating

Continual reassessment of pain is:

- essential if there is no early improvement in pain
- helpful in guiding a reduction of analgesia

Katie was prescribed paracetamol and codeine phosphate six-hourly and diclofenac eight-hourly. Although Katie admitted that she was reluctant to take medicines, she was reassured by her GP that all the 'pain-killers' worked in different ways and that their effect was additive. Because of her previous history of gastric ulceration she was also prescribed a proton pump inhibitor to protect her from the effects of the diclofenac. She was also prescribed a two day course of diazepam six-hourly to relieve the muscle spasm. Katie was encouraged to mobilize gently and to take warm showers. She was encouraged to place a warm or cold pack beneath her lower back to see if either brought relief.

Katie was told to contact her GP immediately if she had any problems with micturating or if she developed leg pain. She was also told to contact her GP again in two days when she had finished the course of diazepam if the pain was not significantly better.

The importance of taking the prescribed medications regularly was emphasized. Katie was advised to gradually reduce her analgesia as her pain decreased rather than stopping all medications at the same time. Katie followed these instructions and her pain score decreased to 4/10 after the first doses of medications. By the end of the week she had stopped all medication and accepted a mild continual backache (pain score 2/10).

Three weeks later Katie developed severe sciatica in both legs. Between episodes of pain (pain score of 10/10) she was pain-free but was terrified of moving in case she precipitated pain. She had taken paracetamol, codeine and diclofenac that she had left over from the treatment of her back pain but these had not helped her sciatica.

Her GP explained the cause of her pain and explained that nerve pain might not be responsive to anti-inflammatory agents and opioids. Instead Katie's GP recommended 10mg amitriptyline to be taken at night, since, unlike its antidepressant effect that may take some weeks to provide any benefit, amitriptyline can be effective at reducing neuropathic pain within a few hours in some patients. Katie was reassured that the majority of cases of sciatica resolved spontaneously but it was emphasized that if she developed increased pain or any bladder problems she must seek immediate medical advice.

Katie felt some improvement in her sciatica following the amitriptyline but the following day her legs were numb and she had developed bilateral foot drop. She also realized that she had not micturated for 12h. Katie's GP confirmed acute urinary retention and arranged for Katie's emergency admission to a neurosurgical unit. Urgent magnetic resonance imaging (MRI) confirmed a central disc prolapse with neural compression and Katie had an emergency discectomy within four hours of admission to prevent permanent neurological deficit. On awakening she had immediate relief from her leg symptoms, and bladder function returned to normal after two days.

3.3 **Summary**

- Clear explanations help reassure and can assist compliance.
- Using pain scores can help guide therapy and be an objective measure of improvement.
- Persistent pain should be reassessed regularly so that clinical changes are noticed.
- Simple analgesia given regularly is usually more effective than intermittently for a persistent pain.
- Using analgesic agents from different classes can help treat severe pain.
- Neuropathic pain may respond better to drugs that are not routinely used for pain, e.g. antidepressants or anti-epileptic agents.
- It is important to be attentive to the development of serious pathology.

Chapter 4

Some treatments cause chronic pain: can we reduce the risk?

Brigitta Brandner

For many, the million dollar question is whether chronic pain can be prevented. In the opening chapter of this book some of the determinants of chronic pain were discussed. Many of them relate to psychosocial issues that play a part in the development of pretty much all major Western ailments. They are tied in to a person's life, work and relationships and become very difficult to unravel without effort at a national level. This chapter looks at the pains that doctors can cause. Surgery and trauma are potent stimulators of pain and sometimes this persists. We will explore possible strategies to prevent chronic pain from developing in a patient undergoing a lower limb amputation, which is a common and distressing experience for amputees.

4.1 Terry's ischaemic leg pain

Terry is a 55-year-old lorry driver who has smoked all his life. He used to suffer calf pain when he walked any distance but this has become worse and now he has constant unremitting leg and foot pain. In the past he has lost the tips of some of his toes because of inadequate blood flow. He hasn't had a good night's sleep in months. Recently he was admitted to hospital and the vascular surgeon is discussing his suitability for a bypass operation to improve blood flow to his leg. Several investigations need to be undertaken before a decision can be made.

Initial analgesia

Terry is referred to the acute pain team in the hospital on the day of his admission. His GP and his surgeon have been struggling to find effective analgesia for his escalating pain just before he came in. The World Health Organizations' ladder of analgesia is a good starting point: Terry has already been prescribed regular paracetamol and diclofenac in combination and when he came into hospital he was taking these. He is able to report that weak opioids (such as dihydrocodeine and tramadol) were started six months ago and were useful, but have not been touching his pain recently. The pain team start immediate-release morphine when they meet Terry. Over his first week in hospital they add up the amount of morphine he uses on a daily basis to control his pain. They use this sum to set the dose and switch him to modified-release, twice-daily morphine with immediate-release morphine for any breakthrough pain. He has begun to sleep much better and generally looks much calmer and less troubled than when he was first admitted.

Unfortunately for Terry, medical, surgical and radiological treatment does not help his limb perfusion and the vascular team explain to him that they feel his leg should be amputated. He acknowledges that the drugs he is taking are causing considerable side-effects as he is sleepy all the time and having hallucinations. He is unable to cooperate with physiotherapy and his pain is becoming worse so he is keen to go ahead with the amputation.

Often patients at this stage assume that surgery will 'take all pain away' and it is essential that Terry is informed about phantom limb and postsurgical pain. If his expectations are not managed preoperatively and he is left with residual pain, his recovery in both physical and mental terms will be hard and possibly never complete with a very difficult situation to manage in the community.

- **Phantom limb pain** is very distressing and up to 80% of amputees can suffer from phantom limb pain at some stage
- The non-existent limb is painful and often feels like it is fixed in a certain position
- The pain is commonly of a shooting and burning nature
- Severe preoperative pain can result in increased postoperative phantom limb pain, so every effort should be made to achieve adequate pain relief before surgery

Pre-emptive analgesia

The idea that you can 'nip something in the bud' to prevent or postpone an untoward outcome is not new. Like pensions, investing in good health in one's early decades can stand you in good stead later on. The concept of pre-emptive analgesia, i.e. to treat pain before the noxious stimuli starts, has been of great interest to pain physicians over the last two decades. The idea is to block pain transmission so that central sensitization does not occur (see Chapter 2) and cause irreversible changes in the central nervous system.

With this in mind, starting an epidural for analgesia 72h preoperatively has shown a reduction in the frequency of phantom limb pain in the early postoperative period; unfortunately these effects are not maintained after six months. Nevertheless, it will significantly improve the patient's experience of disfiguring surgery.

Terry opted to have an elective preoperative epidural sited and was given a mixture of local anaesthetic and opioids through it. His oral pain relief drugs were no longer required and he felt much more alert without any nausea. Terry's pain was well controlled in the days running up to his operation.

Perioperative management

Terry's epidural anaesthesia and analgesia were continued through his operation; he had a light general anaesthetic in addition to the regional technique. If regional anaesthesia had been contraindicated for him, local nerve infiltration could have been used to prevent the acute nerve excitation associated with cutting the major nerves.

Postoperative management

After Terry's operation his epidural analgesia is continued and opioid side-effects, such as nausea, respiratory depression and constipation, are thus minimized. If he didn't have an epidural, strong opioids would have been given by the intravenous route using a patient-controlled analgesia system along with other modes of analgesia.

Ongoing pain

Clinicians are increasingly aware that pain can persist after surgery. The statistics regarding its prevalence make interesting reading and should be taken into account when surgery is being considered:

- breast surgery 11–49%
- cholecystectomy 3–56%
- inguinal herniorraphy 0–63%
- vasectomy 0–37%
- thoracotomy 5–67%

About 17% of all patients presenting to a chronic pain clinic recall surgery as the main causal event. This is particularly common after surgery that causes nerve injury, as in Terry's case. Once the changes have been manifested they can be difficult to treat and long-lasting changes occur. Three days after his operation, Terry starts to complain about severe shooting pain where his leg used to be. There are a number of important pathophysiological processes that might be involved. These can lead to permanent pain.

The pain that Terry describes sounds neuropathic, i.e. pain-initiated or caused by a primary lesion or dysfunction in the nervous system. **Terms that people often use to describe neuropathic pain are: burning, shooting, electric, bursting and tight**. Neuropathic pain can start in the first week after surgery but it can start much later. Pain still present six months after surgery is likely to persist. Terry agrees to try a drug that may help neuropathic pain. A useful concept is numbers-needed-to-treat (NNT): the number of patients who need to be treated to achieve 50% reduction of pain in one patient.

- **Peripheral sensitization**: the traumatized area will painful due to local mediators causing erythema and oedema
- **Central sensitization**: this ongoing process will increase the receptive area in the spinal cord and therefore the peripheral area of increased pain will be larger than the area traumatized by surgery
- **Allodynia**: as a result of nervous system changes, simple touch will cause a painful reaction
- **Anatomical and genetic changes**: once started, these can be irreversible and cause a memory of processes that maintain pain

Numbers needed to treat for neuropathic pain	
• amitriptyline	2.4
• gabapentin	3.7
• carbamazepine	3.3
• selective serotonin reuptake inhibitors	6.7

Terry has nightmares with amitriptyline. He is changed to gabapentin and tolerates a dose of 600mg three times a day very well. He reports less frequency of his shooting pain and his sleep has improved.

There are a few studies available about early treatment with neuropathic agents: a 50% reduction in pain prevalence has been achieved at six months with the use of low-dose amitriptyline early in the treatment of shingles; and pre-emptive gabapentin has reduced the severity of postoperative pain in mastectomy patients. There are no studies yet about the use of gabapentin before limb amputation to reduce phantom limb pain.

Treatment after discharge

It is important to convey honestly the possible outcomes of surgery and explain that phantom pain is a frequent occurrence after an amputation; some people who have had breast surgery report phantom symptoms too. Neuropathic pain has a tendency to improve, but if it persists longer than 6–12 months it is likely to be more difficult to alleviate. Treating neuropathic pain has greater success if started early. Neuropathic agents can be reduced after the patient had been controlled for 6–12 weeks to see if they are still required. If at any stage the pain becomes worse, other factors should be excluded such as local infection or a stump neuroma.

Transcutaneous electrical nerve stimulation (TENS), acupuncture, spinal cord stimulation and cognitive–behavioural treatments can all be considered for the treatment of persistent phantom limb pain.

4.2 Summary

- Ongoing pain after surgery has to be diagnosed and treated promptly.
- Phantom limb pain is a very distressing, chronic, postsurgical pain.
- The analgesic ladder is a useful approach to good analgesia.
- Chronic pain after surgery is often due to nerve injury and drugs used for neuropathic pain should be considered.

Bibliography

Bach, S., Noreng, M.F., and Tjellden, N.U. (1998). Phantom limb pain in amputees during the first 12 months following limb amputation, after pre-operative lumbar epidural blockade. *Pain* **33**(3), 297–301.

Sindrup, S.H. and Jensen, T.S. (1999). Efficacy of pharmacological treatments of neuropathic pain: an update and effect related to mechanism of drug action. *Pain* **83**(3), 389–400.

Wilson, J.A., Colvin, L.A., and Power, I. (2002). Acute neuropathic pain after surgery. *R. Coll. Anaesth. Bull.* **15**, 739–743.

Chapter 5

Assessing people with long-standing pain

Andrew Souter

Assessing patients properly is a crucial first step in medicine. Faced with someone who has had long-term pain, the first response is to do anything to avoid being pulled into a long and difficult conversation. Often these patients will already be very familiar and perhaps it is felt that nothing new will emerge, or no progress will be made. However, a simple assessment in the form of history and examination will point the way to appropriate management. Firstly there are treatments that can be provided in primary care; and secondly, because of waiting lists in all parts of the health service, the best referral is one that goes to the right specialist who has the necessary information on first seeing the patient.

5.1 The history

- Did the pain start following an incident, and when did it start?
- *Site and radiation.* Spinal pain may be referred peripherally. While the pain may be in the distribution of a dermatome, this is often not the case.
- *Character.* Neuropathic pain is described in unusual terms such as burning, sensitive, electric, bursting, tight or like pins and needles. This may distinguish it from inflammatory or nociceptive pain.
- *Timing.* Is the pain continuous or intermittent; is it mechanical, does it relate to posture? Neuropathic pain may be unrelated to stimulus, or it may be lancinating.
- *Aggravating and relieving factors.* Excessive bed rest rarely gives relief in chronic musculoskeletal pain. Musculoskeletal pain is often intermittent and is precipitated by particular movements or situations, e.g. walking, standing or sitting.

5.2 Psychological factors

Chronic pain rarely appears alone. Psychological distress is commonplace and should be enquired about early in the assessment. Anxiety, depression, anger and withdrawal from family and friends can have an impact on the severity of the pain and the ability to recover and respond to treatment. A common feature of these patients is a need to be believed and taken seriously. Attitudes and beliefs regarding the meaning of the pain may hinder rehabilitation; chronic musculoskeletal pain rarely needs rest; this may be counter-intuitive for some patients.

5.3 Social factors

Work and family life can both affect and be affected by chronic pain. Injury and chronic pain can lead to loss of work. Litigation, common today in workplace and other injuries, will have a bearing on the attitude of the patient to chronic pain and the ability to recover from it.

5.4 Previous investigations and treatment

It is pointless repeating investigations unless symptoms and signs have changed although occasionally the ability of the patient to accept a diagnosis and progress with treatment may be hindered until further investigation is carried out. Likewise, it is not appropriate to refer for more treatment such as physiotherapy where this has previously been unhelpful.

5.5 Red Flags in people with back pain

Acute spinal cord or cauda equina lesions need immediate referral and investigation. History of incontinence, limb weakness or saddle anaesthesia must not be ignored. Other red flags for serious spinal pathology requiring review by a specialist who is able to see patients urgently include: presentation under the age of 20 years or onset over 55 years; non-mechanical pain; thoracic pain; a past history of relevant conditions (carcinoma, steroids, HIV); people who are unwell, or have weight loss; widespread neurological symptoms or signs; and structural deformity.

5.6 Simon's shoulder pain

History. Simon is 53-years-old, right-handed, and complains of a two year history of pain in his right shoulder that may have come on after a rare game of tennis.

Site and radiation. The pain is strongest around his shoulder, associated with neck pain and radiates down his arm. Pain originating from the spine may refer to lateral structures. Pain radiating down the arm into the hand suggests cervical radiculopathy. This 'red flag' needs further assessment with a neurological examination.

Character. On direct questioning he has had some burning and tingling pain in the forearm which points to a neuropathic pain of radiculopathy. However, this resolved soon after his pain began two years ago.

Timing. Simon has a continuous background of pain, but whenever he moves his shoulder his pain is much worse. Pain arising from the shoulder joint is often mechanical. Pain from the cervical spine may give a more constant referred pain in the shoulder region.

Other factors. Simon is a draughtsman and finds that the pain makes it difficult to concentrate on technical drawings. You need to find out about the current work situation and life outside work. You should enquire about a history of trauma or whiplash.

Examination. This will be directed by the history. Although in chronic musculoskeletal pain examination is often unrewarding, it does send positive signals to the patients regarding your commitment to their problem.

Neurological examination. Where there is spinal pain with radiation, abnormal neurological signs such as loss of muscle power, sensation or reflexes should be excluded. The neurology of the lower limbs should always be examined in patients with neck pain. The presence of these so-called 'red flags' warrants urgent referral and investigation.

General examination. Other 'red flags' in examination include spinal deformity, e.g. scoliosis, kyphosis and the presence of other major pathology such as cancers or infections.

Examining Simon, it appears that there are no abnormal neurological signs, although there is a history that there was transient nerve impingement. His pain is confined to the shoulder with tension radiating to his arm and neck. As he has tried a course of physiotherapy and has worked his way through a catalogue of analgesia, you decide to refer him to a shoulder surgeon for an opinion.

5.7 **Fatimah's bad back**

History. Fatimah has had three months of low back pain; she is 72-years-old. She also has pain radiating to her left ankle. She had breast cancer successfully treated two years ago and is otherwise well with no weight loss or night sweats.

Examination. Fatimah has muscle spasm in her lumbar paraspinal muscles which is worse on the right side. She finds it very difficult to bend forwards as her back pain is worse and bending sends shooting sensations down her right leg. Severely restricted movements and/or tenderness may predict spinal pathology.

Neurology. Although the examination is limited by her pain, there does not appear to be any alteration of Fatimah's reflexes. She has some reduced sensation over pretty much the whole of her foot and dorsiflexion of her great toe is weak. Perineal sensation should be tested to exclude a cauda equina lesion. Lower limb weakness, loss of sensation or reflex predict a nerve root lesion and these need urgent further specialist assessment.

General features. Recurrence of breast cancer should be sought. Cachexia, anaemia, abscesses, fever and other features are suggestive of serious pathology and should also be excluded.

There are several worrying features in Fatimah's history and she should be referred to a spinal surgeon for assessment: a history of cancer, nerve involvement with back pain and her age are all 'red flags'.

5.8 The pain clinic

The pain clinic has a range of roles to play. Patients are usually sent here following assessment by a specialist. After this, an in-depth assessment of psychosocial factors can lead to multidisciplinary approach to helping people in long-term pain. On the medical side, targeted local anaesthetic blocks can delineate more clearly the site of origin of the pain where there is a diagnostic dilemma. For example, nerve-root blocks can determine which nerve root is giving rise to radicular pain or cervical facet joint blocks can determine whether shoulder pain is coming from the posterior structures in the neck or the shoulder itself. The skills of the pain clinic will depend on your local provider: they will be able to tell you what they can provide.

Key points

- A full pain history is helpful in diagnosis.
- Psychosocial factors affect, and are affected by, chronic pain.
- A psychosocial history should be elicited early.
- 'Red flags' in history and examination need urgent investigation.
- The local pain clinic is useful in further assessment and treatment.

Chapter 6

Injections, invasive treatments and the 'whole patient' view

John Lee

This chapter discusses the care of a patient who is being managed in a disjointed fashion. It describes a complex patient with a standard back pain problem where a failure of effective communication leads to an unhappy customer and a disgruntled and bewildered family. It draws on this experience to show how teams like the pain service can occasionally work to improve collaboration and communication. It also describes the medical treatments that pain clinics may offer.

John is a 63-year-old with end stage renal failure from hypertensive renal disease. His life is dependent on renal replacement therapy from haemodialysis. He has had problems with vascular access for his dialysis, and he currently has a tunnelled synthetic access catheter to a great vein.

John now develops severe back pain that radiates down his right leg to his calf. He is referred to the pain management team. When questioned closely, he appears to have both mechanical back pain and sciatic pain. A magnetic resonance imaging (MRI) scan reveals that he has both degeneration of his lumbar facet joints and bilateral compression of nerve roots at the L5/S1 intervertebral foramina.

John underwent facet joint injections a few weeks later. His pain was much improved but he was left with residual sciatic type discomfort and he was scheduled for root nerve blocks at the lumbosacral level.

Unfortunately, he became gravely unwell with septicaemia due to an infected intravascular catheter. Following his recovery and after a spell on ITU, his back was more painful and the pain team requested further imaging. New MRI pictures suggested that there was infection involving his intervertebral discs and he was referred to the orthopaedic surgeons who recommended a long course of antibiotics.

Patterns of back pain

Facet joint pain:
- worse with rotation, lateral flexion and extension of the spine

Discogenic pain
- localized low back pain
- associated back muscle spasm
- worse with sitting and forward flexion

Nerve root pain
- unilateral leg pain worse than low back pain
- radiates in a dermatomal pattern
- typical neuropathic description of pain
  - burning
  - bursting
  - electrical
  - shooting
  - tight
- localized signs, e.g. abnormal sensation, altered reflexes, muscle weakness
- straight leg raising may exacerbate leg pain

Over the next few months, John's pain was managed with a number of different medications with variable success. As he had both neuropathic and mechanical pain, agents working on both of these paths were appropriate. There is always a concern about using drugs in people that are dialysis dependent, as many drugs (or their metabolites) can build up to toxic levels. Communication between the renal, pain and orthopaedic teams was largely through the ward nursing staff, the specialist pain nurse and writing in the medical notes. Gabapentin was suggested to the renal physicians by the pain team (using a small dose given after his dialysis). Tramadol was also prescribed, and then a small dose of morphine was added. Some time during the weeks of his escalating requirements for pain relief, John began to become confused. The pain team nurse was contacted by the renal physicians as it was felt this was due to the drugs for his pain. In the interim, the renal physicians stopped these three new medications. John's confusion settled, and he was restarted on morphine by the pain team in the form of morphine sulphate tablets (MSTs) with immediate-release morphine for breakthrough with a total daily dose of any form of morphine at approximately 30mg. The morphine was partially helpful for his pain but unfortunately over the next few weeks, John became increasingly sedated and confused. This became such an issue that all medications were again stopped, and the pain team asked if the physicians would examine other medical causes of confusion: John is known to have ischaemic

Common pain clinic injections

Injections:

- fairly superficial; X-rays usually not used to localize
  - muscular tender points
  - suprascapular nerve (for shoulder pain)
  - inguinal field block
  - lateral femoral cutaneous nerve
  - greater occipital nerve (base of skull)
- deep; X-rays usually used to localize
  - facet joints
  - epidural space
  - thoracic paravertebral region
  - nerve roots as they exit the spinal cord
  - lumbar sympathetic plexus
  - coeliac plexus
- others
  - intravenous regional guanethidine block
  - stellate ganglion block

Other pain clinic interventions:

- pain-specific drug therapy
  - drug challenges with receptor-specific antagonists, e.g. lidocaine, ketamine or phentolamine
  - anticonvulsants, antidepressants or other unusual drugs
  - advising and managing the use of opioids in chronic pain
- specialist clinics
  - physiotherapy for long-term pain
  - psychology for long-term pain
  - acupuncture
  - research projects
- pain management programmes (multiprofessional structured programmes encouraging self-management using cognitive behavioural methods)

heart disease, and other infective or cerebrovascular causes of confusion were a distinct possibility. His morphine was exchanged for oxycodone, as changing opioids is sometimes helpful with adverse side-effects; morphine and its metabolites can also accumulate in renal disease with toxic effects. The oxycodone was better tolerated, but some of John's neuropathic pain persisted.

During the course of the four months when John was cared for as an outpatient, his family were expressing increasing dissatisfaction with the hospital services through the nursing staff: the family were at work at ward round times. They felt that clinicians were not addressing John's pain adequately. His wife also felt that their GP left John's medical care up to the renal physicians, who expressed their view to the pain team that they were only providing care for his renal replacement. John himself often reported that he was 'fine' when seen by the pain team around the time of his dialysis, only to keep his working wife up all nights of the weekend with him complaining of pain. John was repeatedly staying in hospital after his dialysis to manage his symptoms. Eventually, the renal team requested a case conference with John, his wife, orthopaedic team and the pain team.

On the day of the case conference, the only member of staff to turn up was the Consultant in Pain Medicine. A ward nurse was able to join the meeting with John and his wife. The Senior House Officer from the renal team who arranged the meeting was on annual leave, and no one else was free. John's wife was angry because she felt she had been kept poorly informed by the doctors. She felt that the different groups of doctors did not appear to be communicating with each other about John's problems. The family found the meeting helpful because the pain team was able to go through John's medical conditions in relation to his symptoms, and discuss why there had been difficulties about getting both the type and dose of medication correct for him. He and his family were also given very clear instructions about the use of his pain drugs. John was able to spend more time at home between dialysis sessions following this case conference.

Managing patients with long-term pain relies on many different groups

- The patient and their carers/loved ones
- GPs and the primary care teams
- Hospital experts
    - local to the patient
    - specialist centres further afield

Lines of responsibility should be clear, and the GP should remain fully informed as the patient's linchpin.

John went on to tolerate a smaller dose of gabapentin, and after an interval of around eight months on antibiotics, underwent a spinal fusion which greatly improved his back pain.

One of the greatest complaints against doctors is that they communicate poorly, and this is an issue not only between doctor and patient, but also amongst hospital specialists and between them and their colleagues in primary care. The collective responsibility of his carers should have provided:

1. Better team-working to maximize the skills of a multiprofessional group rather than relying on one area or another to take responsibility.
2. Better communication both to the patient, his family, and between the providers of care.
3. A coherent voice and message from his medical carers. There has been a tendency with increasing specialization for professionals to speak with different voices and to appear fragmented. This probably cost John time in arriving at the best path for his care because problems were being thrown backwards and forwards around a loop.

John's case has also shown how a range of treatments may help with pain as a careful history will often suggest different causes for pain and discomfort.

Reference

Calman, K. (1994). The profession of medicine. *Br. Med. J.* **309**, 1140–1143.

Chapter 7

What should I feel like after treatment at the pain clinic?

Simon Dolin and Lucy Ward

Patients who have been to the pain clinic may run into trouble as a consequence of the treatments provided. They may be unhappy about seeking advice from the pain clinic if they feel worse after the treatment, or they may contact their GP surgery first. This chapter will discuss the management of a patient with lower back pain (LBP) and the possible complications that a GP may be asked for help with.

Lower back pain is a common problem with a great deal of disability and many days lost from work. There are a number of procedures and therapies performed in the pain clinic that may help sufferers improve their functional ability. These are best accompanied by a gradual increase in exercise, activity and stretching, alongside patient education to help to prevent recurrence. Each clinic will have a different set-up directed to accomplishing this aim.

As with all therapies, there may be complications that arise after pain clinic procedures. Most are minor with severe complications being uncommon. Invasive procedures have general risks and specific risks. Some of the general complications may have serious consequences that need rapid action: for example, a deep-sited infection or haematoma may give rise to neural compromise and needs prompt and effective emergency treatment. Specific complications are discussed under the relevant intervention.

General complications of invasive procedures

- allergy to some component
- bruising
- bleeding
- infection (deep or superficial)
- worse pain
- lack of success

7.1 TENS (transcutaneous electrical nerve stimulation)

TENS is the passage of a small modulated electrical current between two adhesive surface electrodes placed on the skin of the painful area. It can be effective in controlling some LBP and many patients will try a TENS machine at some point. The pads are placed over the area of pain, and the patient adjusts the pulse rate and amplitude according to effect.

Problems encountered include:

- difficulty placing the pads
- skin irritation and scorching under the pads
- muscle contractions during use

TENS is probably best avoided with a pacemaker but this can be discussed with the patient's cardiologist. The pads should not be applied over a numb area as this may result in burns.

7.2 Acupuncture

This is performed in many pain clinics, and has been found to be of some use in LBP. Improvement is short or medium term and repeated treatments may be necessary. As with many interventions, it may provide a window of pain relief during which time exercises and stretches can cause a longer-term improvement in the underlying condition and the maintainers of pain.

Possible side-effects are:

- temporary exacerbation of pain (common)
- short-lived nausea and tiredness (common)
- local infection
- nerve or blood vessel damage
- pneumothorax if needles placed near the chest wall (rare)
- cardiac tamponade if needles placed over heart (rare)

7.3 Epidural injections

These are usually performed in a patient who exhibits signs and symptoms of nerve root pain (sciatica). They are normally a combination of local anaesthetic (lignocaine or bupivacaine) and steroid (methylprednisolone as Depomedrone, or triamcinolone as Kenalog) injected in the lumbar region and can be performed under X-ray guidance. Complications of epidural injections may be immediate, early or late. (Complications of steroid injections are described in Section 7.6.)

Immediate problems:

- hypotension—occurs immediately and resolves early (common)
- leg weakness and numbness—resolves within hours and the patient is only discharged when they can walk safely (common)
- localized pain may occur during the injection and for a few days afterwards (common)
- inadvertent spinal block will cause total paralysis and the patient will be treated in hospital until the effects have resolved (rare)
- inadvertent intravascular injection with convulsions (rare)
- risk of spinal cord damage (rare)

Post dural-puncture headache, an early problem:

This occurs if there is accidental puncture of the dura mater resulting in a cerebrospinal fluid leak. The incidence is around 1 in 100 cases although is probably less in clinicians with more experience. It classically occurs 1–2 days after the procedure, is postural, fronto-occipital and exacerbated by sudden movements or straining. A patient who presents with this picture after an epidural should be referred back to the clinician who performed the procedure for further management, and may need to be admitted to hospital for an epidural blood patch (using the patient's own blood).

Late complications:

Epidural abscess or haematoma. These complications are extremely rare, but may present with persistent pyrexia, back pain and evidence of spinal cord compression such as leg weakness, and incontinence. If it occurs, the patient should be referred as an emergency to a neurosurgeon for surgical decompression, as permanent damage can occur with any delay.

7.4 Facet joint injections or denervation

These procedures are performed for patients with pain arising from lumbar facet joints. Pain is typically worse with rotation, lateral flexion and extension of the back. Whether the joint is injected with local anaesthetic and steroid, or undergoes radiofrequency denervation will depend on local practice and expertise. Injection with local anaesthetic and steroid may result in epidural spread of the injectate, and therefore any of the complications discussed above.

Complications of radiofrequency lesioning of the nerve supplying the facet joint include:

- postoperative pain (common, and should diminish over a week)
- cutaneous numbness (rarely)
- dysaesthesia (rare unpleasant cutaneous sensations)

- anaesthesia dolorosa (rare pain in an area of skin that has no sensation)

If any of the above occur and are persistent, the patient should be referred back to the pain clinic.

7.5 Intradiscal treatment

These are used in patients with pain arising specifically from the lumbar intervertebral discs which are thought to account for up to 40% of back pain. Painful discs can be diagnosed by low-pressure discography assisted by magnetic resonance imaging. An abnormal and painful disc can be treated by placing an electrode in the disc for intradiscal electrotherapy (IDET). Availability of treatment will be limited by local expertise and practice.

Complications are not common but include:

- vascular injury
- discitis
- subdural empyema
- spinal cord injury
- prevertebral abscess

If any of these complications are suspected the patient should be referred back to the clinician who performed the procedure.

7.6 Steroid injections

Most of the injections described above include the use of steroid. This is usually in the form of a depot preparation in order to prolong activity, and each preparation has a different propensity to cause systemic effects.

Side-effects include:

- insomnia
- flushing
- mood changes (uncommon)
- hyperglycaemia in diabetics (uncommon)
- pituitary suppression (rare, especially for infrequent injections)

If the patient experiences these effects, the symptoms are likely to settle spontaneously. If blood sugar control is worsened this should be managed as appropriate, remembering that once the steroid effect resolves, sugar control should return to previous levels.

7.7 **Pain management programmes (PMPs)**

These are aimed at improving the patient's quality of life, and involve a team approach to education, goal setting, pacing of activities, coping strategies, drug withdrawal if possible, and general fitness. They occur on either an outpatient or inpatient basis as a group activity. There is good evidence for the effectiveness of PMPs. The evidence for repeating programmes is weak and is therefore unlikely to be justified.

7.8 **Summary**

There are a number of different procedures performed by the pain management specialist for LBP, and each procedure will have complications due to both the procedure itself and due to what is injected. Although most of these complications are rare, some are serious and can lead to significant morbidity. These should be diagnosed and treated appropriately.

Bibliography

Dolin, S. and Padfield, N. (2003). *Pain Medicine Manual.* Elsevir.

Grady, K.M. *et al.* (1997). *Key Topics in Chronic Pain.* BIOS Scientific Publishers.

Lord, S. *et al.* (2002). Radiofrequency procedures in chronic pain. *Best Pract. Res. Clin. Anaesthesiol.* **16**, 597–617.

Chapter 8

Prescribing for people with pain originating in the nervous system. Part 1. Tricyclic antidepressants

Simon Davies

This is the first of two chapters describing how drugs which are not usually classed as analgesics can be used to treat neuropathic pain. Chapter 8 is about tricyclic antidepressants (TCAs) and Chapter 9 about anticonvulsants. There is also a table which suggests how the drugs can be prescribed.

8.1 Fatima's sprained ankle

A 59-year-old woman has sprained her ankle, and despite having had a course of physiotherapy, continues to suffer pain. Two months after her accident, she also describes swelling of her ankle, and the ankle going 'hot and cold'. The ankle is particularly troublesome at night, keeping her awake. Her GP prescribes amitriptyline 25mg at night, increasing in steps to 75mg, which greatly improves her pain and the quality of her sleep. This does improve her symptoms but because of their odd nature, she is referred to the orthopaedic surgeons for an opinion. The consultant feels there is no bone damage and that she has an element of complex regional pain syndrome; he encourages her to continue with the exercises taught by the physiotherapist and reassures her.

Complex regional pain syndrome

- often results from a relatively minor soft tissue injury (type I)
- can also be associated with peripheral nerve damage (type II)
- is a form of neuropathic pain
- is associated with regional abnormalities
  - swelling
  - sweating

Six months later, her symptoms are much reduced and she is discharged from the orthopaedic surgeon's clinic. She is advised that if symptoms become more troublesome she may benefit from seeing a chronic pain specialist.

8.2 Discussion

Antidepressants have been used to treat a wide variety of neuropathic pain for over 40 years. While the treatment of neuropathic pain remains an unlicensed indication for many antidepressants in the UK, they are drugs with which all GPs have experience and for which the use beyond the product licence is widely supported.

The efficacy of antidepressants has been shown in a number of trials and supported by meta-analysis. Most work supports the use of TCAs and they are generally considered to be of more use than selective serotonin reuptake inhibitors (SSRIs). A number needed to treat (NNT) of 2.9 [95% confidence interval(CI) 2.4–3.7] to gain 50% pain relief was calculated from a meta-analysis of trials using TCAs in patients with mixed types of neuropathic pain. Unfortunately there is not enough evidence to suggest which TCA is the best, but most experience rests with amitriptyline. Results from the same review gave NNTs for SSRIs of between 5 and 15 (although the number of patients was much smaller). There have also been some positive trials for newer antidepressants such as venlafaxine and duloxetine (now approved in the UK for the treatment of diabetic neuropathy).

Antidepressants mainly act through blocking the reuptake of serotonin and/or noradrenaline in the spinal cord where these chemicals have an inhibitory effect on pain transmission. Amitriptyline also has effects on sodium channels, acetylcholine receptors and *n*-methyl-d-aspartate (NMDA) receptors, all of which are important in the pathophysiology of neuropathic pain.

The classical indication of when an antidepressant may be useful is if the patient complains of burning pain (using anticonvulsants for shooting pains). This is now considered to be untrue and it is probably worth using antidepressants in all types of neuropathic pain.

One of the main benefits of TCAs is the improvement in sleep seen with its sedative action and this should be exploited in the timing of administration of the drug. The effects of antidepressants in neuropathic pain appear to be independent of their effects on mood although an improvement in mood may be a useful adjunct. The speed of onset is usually faster (1–7 days) and effective doses are usually lower (25–150mg amitriptyline per day) than as an antidepressant used for depression. It is very important that patients should be made aware that these drugs are being given for their pain and not for depression.

Antidepressants have a variety of unwanted effects, the most problematic of which is often excessive sedation. They also have a number of effects relating to their anticholinergic actions (e.g. postural hypotension, dry mouth, urinary retention and a rise in intraocular pressure, and should be avoided in people with closed angle glaucoma). Unfortunately many patients who have neuropathic pain are elderly where these side-effects are even more troublesome. The same review as above gave the number needed to harm for minor and major side-effects for all antidepressants as 3.7 (CI 2.9–5.2) and 22 (13.5–58) respectively.

By giving the drug at night, starting at a low dose (e.g. amitriptyline 10mg) and increasing the dose slowly (e.g. by 10–25mg per week) some of these side-effects can be avoided. If excessive daytime drowsiness is seen, then the drug can be given earlier in the evening. The dose of amitriptyline should be increased until pain relief is obtained or until side-effects become intolerable (with a maximum dose of 150mg). If low doses of amitriptyline are not tolerated then it is sometimes worth considering a different tricyclic antidepressant with a different side-effect profile such as imipramine. If patients do not tolerate TCAs then consideration should be given to starting an SSRI, which, even though less efficacious, are generally better tolerated.

There is increasing evidence that the early treatment of neuropathic pain may help to stop the pain becoming a chronic condition. The primary care setting where these patients usually present and where the doctors have experience with prescribing antidepressants is an ideal time to start these drugs. This not only treats the patient earlier, but if the drug is ineffective it may allow more specialized treatment to be started sooner once the patient reaches a pain clinic.

In patients where depression is a significant problem, newer antidepressants will probably be more effective. Drugs such as mirtazapine or venlafaxine may be useful in managing both the pain and the depression. There is some evidence that SSRIs (e.g. paroxetine) should be the drugs of first choice for people with facial pain and post traumatic-stress.

Using amitriptyline in neuropathic pain

- more efficacy for tricyclic antidepressants over others
- 30% patients will have greater than 50% pain relief
- both pain reduction and improvement in sleep quality
- emphasize drug is prescribed for analgesia
- troublesome side-effects: sedation, postural hypotension, dry mouth, urinary retention, blurred vision
- if there are side-effects, maintain the lowest tolerable dose and try increasing more slowly

Start with small dose at night and increase slowly, e.g.

Week no.	Amitriptyline(mg)	Notes
1	10	
2	20	} Consider 25mg tablet
3	30	
4	40	
5	50	Consider 50mg tablet
6	60	
7	70	} Consider 50 + 25mg tablets
8	80	
9	90	
10	100	Consider two 50mg tablets

Dose may be increased to 150mg if useful

Bibliography

Bandolier. The Oxford Pain Internet Site. http://www.jr2.ox.ac.uk/bandolier/booth/painpag/index.html.

Anon. (2000). Drug treatment of neuropathic pain. *Drug Therapeut. Bull*, **38**, 89–93.

Goldstein, D.J., Lu, Y., Detke, M.J., Lee, T.C., and Iyengar, S. (2005). Duloxetine vs. placebo in patients with painful diabetic neuropathy. *Pain*, **116**, 109–118.

McQuay, H.J. and Moore, R.A. (1997). Antidepressants and chronic pain. Effective analgesia in neuropathic pain and other syndromes (Editorial). *B.M.J.* ed. **314**, 763–776.

McQuay, H.J., Tramèr, M., Nye, B.A., Carroll, D., Wiffen, P.J., and Moore, R.A. (1996). A systematic review of antidepressants in neuropathic pain. *Pain*, **68**, 217–227.

Chapter 9

Prescribing for people with pain originating in the nervous system. Part 2. Anticonvulsants

Sam Chong

This chapter describes the use of anticonvulsants in neuropathic pain. The form of neuropathic pain described here is called central post-stroke pain which can be particularly difficult to treat with a patient driven to distraction by the discomfort. The chapter concludes with a suggested prescribing regimen (Table 9.1) and treatment algorithm (Figure 9.1).

9.1 Nadine's facial pain

A 50-year-old right-handed secretary was admitted to hospital with an episode of dizziness and pain on the left side of her face. The symptoms came on abruptly when she sat down. After this she quickly became nauseated and was falling to the right when walking. She was admitted to hospital and it was noted that she had left facial asymmetry with sensory loss on the same side and right-sided clumsiness. There was no sensory loss in her limbs.

A computed tomography (CT) brain scan showed an area of low attenuation in the right cerebellum with a hint of signal change in the right brainstem consistent with a right-sided brainstem and cerebellar stroke. She had a number of risk factors predisposing her for the stroke: she smoked 40 cigarettes a day and had untreated hypertension. She went on to have a magnetic resonance imaging (MRI) scan of her head which confirmed a stroke involving the right cerebellar hemisphere with damage to the right pons consistent with blockage of a small pontine artery.

She recovered from her ataxia and clumsiness but continued to suffer with severe pain in the left side of her face. The initial 'numb' pain began spreading approximately six months after her stroke, so that it radiated to the left frontal region, into the left temple and across her mouth. She also described a continuous sharp stabbing

Table 9.1 Prescribing regimen for central neuropathic pain

Central neuropathic pain:

- is difficult to treat
- may be delayed after a stroke and it can actually become worse in the absence of new central nervous system damage
- the mainstay of pharmacotherapy are tricyclic antidepressants and anticonvulsants
- combining pharmacotherapy, physiotherapy and psychological techniques may be useful in helping patients to manage their pain

Gabapentin and pregabalin are licensed for use in neuropathic pain. People who are sensitive to side-effects may appreciate a rising dose over six weeks, but some will tolerate this for more than one week. Tablets and capsules are available in a range of doses.

Interval: may be days or weeks	Gabapentin dose (mg)		
	Morning	Afternoon	Evening
1	0	0	300
2	300	0	300
3	300	300	300
4	300	300	600
5	600	300	600
6	600	600	600

Pregabalin is also licensed for neuropathic pain and a simple dosing regimen is available.

Weekly intervals	Pregabalin dose (mg)	
	Morning	Evening
1	75	75
2	150	150
3	300	300

Carbamazepine may be a useful drug in neuropathic pain; practical experience suggests that the side-effects are more problematic. Monitoring of liver function and blood count should be considered.

Weeks	Carbamazepine dose (mg)		
	Morning	Afternoon	Evening
1	100	0	100
2	200	0	200
3	200	200	200

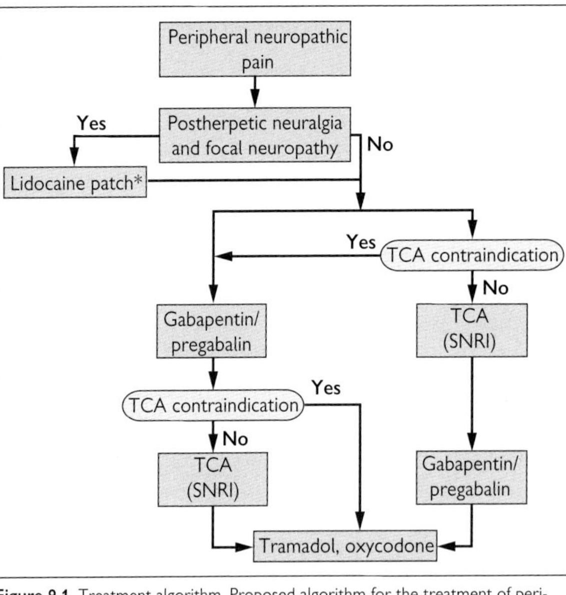

Figure 9.1 Treatment algorithm. Proposed algorithm for the treatment of peripheral neuropathic pain. TCA, tricyclic antidepressants; SNRI, serotonin noradrenaline reputake inhibitors. * Pain-relieving effect of topical lidocaine has been shown in patients with allodynia. [Reproduced with permission from: Algorithm for neuropathic pain treatment: an evidence based proposal. Finnerup, A., Otto B., McQuay C., Jensen A., and Sindru, P. (2005), *Pain* **118**, 289–305.]

sensation, particularly in her left temple. She was diagnosed as having central post-stroke pain.

Her GP prescribed pain killers which did not help her. She was then given amitriptyline titrated up to 50mg at night (see Chapter 8), but this dose did not really help her symptoms and higher doses made her too drowsy during the day. She was seen by a neurologist who added carbamazepine 200mg three times a day which did not help either. On a 0–10 visual analogue scale, the pain was up to 7 for most of the day.

One year after her stroke she continued to report severe burning pain exacerbated by warmth and touch. Face washing was particularly uncomfortable; regardless of the temperature of the water, any thermal stimulation (water either warmer or colder than body temperature) caused a burning sensation. Pain became the main limiting factor affecting her quality of life. She was beginning to withdraw from things she used to enjoy despite her full physical recovery. For example, she used to be proficient at bowls, playing at county-level competitions, but had given this up because she found that whenever it rained, the raindrops hitting the left side of her face were excruciating.

In an effort to control her pain, her neurologist substituted gabapentin for carbamazepine to her regimen. The dose of gabapentin was slowly weaned up to 1.8g a day, then gradually increased up to 2.7g a day. At the same time the dose of carbamazepine was reduced. When she was reviewed four months after starting gabapentin, she said that the pain was under better control. Pain severity on a visual analogue scale was only 4/10. Unfortunately, she also described side-effects; she had difficulty counting, e.g. while playing card games. It was agreed that the dose of gabapentin should be reduced to 2.1g a day and she stopped the carbamazepine completely. Her pain level remained at 3–4 on the visual analogue scale and she was satisfied with this; she had also come to terms with the fact that there was no 'cure' for her pain, and had begun to take up bowls again so that her pain would not get the better of her.

9.2 **Commentary**

Central pain is a difficult condition to treat and more alarmingly for patients the pain may actually increase in severity with time. Typically, the area of sensory loss extends beyond that for pain. Central pain does not respond to conventional analgesics and tricyclic antidepressant drugs are the treatment of first choice. In one placebo-controlled study, amitriptyline was calculated to have an NNT of 1.7 to reduce central pain by 50% (McQuay *et al.*, 1996). Combined data from studies with other tricyclic antidepressants, clomipramine and nortriptyline, gave an NNT of 2.0 for alleviating central pain (McQuay *et al.*, 1996).

There are for fewer studies of anticonvulsants for treating post-stroke pain, which can be thought of as a subset of all central pain states. In a small placebo-controlled study of carbamazepine versus amitriptyline or placebo, carbamazepine was reported to be superior than placebo but not as effective as amitriptyline (Leijon and Bovie, 1989). There is little information on the use of combination therapy but using anticonvulsants and amitriptyline together appears to be a logical way of alleviating central pain. Whereas there are numerous placebo-controlled studies demonstrating the effectiveness of gabapentin in peripheral neuropathic pain, there have been no placebo-controlled trials; there are numerous case studies reporting the effectiveness of gabapentin for treating central pain. In this patient, gabapentin together with carbamazepine and amitriptyline was partially successful but this regime also caused marked blunting of higher mental function. Often if one form of anticonvulsant is associated with side-effects it is worth considering other anticonvulsants such as pregabalin, phenytoin, sodium valproate or clonazepam—this list is not exhaustive. Close cooperation between patient and doctor is necessary to achieve a successful balance between pain relief and side-effects.

Bibliography

Finnerup, N.B., Otto, M., McQuay, H.J., Jensen T.S., Sindrup, S.H. (2005). Algorithm for neuropathic pain treatment: an evidence based proposal. *Pain*, **3**, 289–305.

McQuay, H.J., Tramer, M., Nye, B.A., Carrell, D., Wiffen, P.J., Moore, R.A. (1996). A systematic review of antidepressants in neuropathic pain. *Pain*, **2**–**3**, 217–27.

Chapter 10

Strong opioids in the treatment of people with non-malignant pain

Jon Francis

Opioids are our most powerful analgesics, but prejudice, ignorance and fear of addiction remain barriers to their use in the treatment of chronic non-cancer pain. Attitudes are changing, as witnessed by an increasingly free use of opioid patches; this has created a new set of issues. Improved understanding is needed widely amongst primary care and hospital physicians about the best use of this group of medicines.

10.1 Danielle's back pain

Danielle, aged 65 years, has had mechanical back pain for 15 years. Surgery five years ago made little difference to her pain. Following further investigation and surgical consultation she was told, 'you have to live with your pain'. She takes two tablets of co-codamol (30/500) when required which reduces her pain by 30%, but only for two hours. She admits to taking more than the maximum daily recommended dose often.

Following assessment in a multidisciplinary pain management clinic, she has a trial of both lumbar facet joint injections and a transcutaneous electrical nerve stimulation (TENS) machine. Unfortunately, neither of these helps her.

10.2 Should strong opioids be considered?

Danielle reports a positive but brief response to weak opioids. The mechanism for her chronic pain is known, and, given the failure of other treatments, consideration of a trial of strong opioid medication is warranted. She has a psychological assessment, paying particular attention to drug, alcohol and psychiatric problems.

10.3 Consent to treatment

When considering the use of strong opioids, full patient consent is essential. Time spent outlining the intended benefit of pain relief and improved function, as well as addressing patient concerns, will empower both doctor and patient. Patients can harbour unfounded prejudices and fears about side-effects, tolerance and addiction.

Strong opioid analgesia is not a treatment for anxiety or depression and should not be used accordingly. Combining analgesia with exercise advice and general encouragement that 'hurt does not mean harm' are as essential here as in any patient suffering chronic pain.

Suitability criteria for consideration of strong opioid analgesia

- persistent pain of known mechanism
- failure to respond to other treatments
- demonstrated opioid responsiveness
- willingness to achieve agreed functional targets
- no significant drug, alcohol or psychiatric problem

10.4 Side-effects

Sedation, nausea, vomiting and itching can occur with the use of strong opioid drugs but frequently improve after a few weeks of use. Careful titration reduces the severity and incidence of common side-effects. Should they persist, changing or 'switching' the opioid drug can sometimes improve side-effects whilst maintaining analgesia.

Constipation is common and tends to persist. Encouragement of adequate oral fluid and fruit intake, as well as the use of simple stool softeners and bowel stimulants, can help.

Serious side-effects can occur in about one percent of patients and include respiratory depression, weight gain and hormonal effects such as reduced sexual function, infertility and adrenal suppression.

10.5 Can patients drive?

Strong opioid drugs do not exclude patients from driving. There is no evidence to suggest that patients taking opioids are more likely to have accidents. Whilst opioid medication can produce cognitive changes, so does living in constant pain, and research suggests that analgesia may improve cognitive function. However, it is prudent to encourage the patient to inform the Driving Vehicle Licensing Authority and their insurer.

10.6 What drug do I use and how do I use it?

Danielle was started on a slow release morphine sulphate tablet (MST) at a dose of 20mg twice daily.

Numerous pharmacological possibilities are available but there is little good-quality medical evidence to suggest that anything is better than morphine. Oral morphine can be administered in modified release preparations which can provide 24h cover with a twice daily dose. Short-acting opioids in tablet or liquid form can be helpful in the initial titration phase when ascertaining dose requirements. Drugs should be given by mouth (injectable opioids have no place in the management of chronic non-malignant pain), and by the clock: a constant dose should be given at regular intervals. The use of short-acting opioids can lead to uncontrolled dose escalation and allow the use of opioids to treat psychological distress; this behaviour may become problematic.

Transdermal patch delivery technology has allowed the development of fentanyl and buprenorphine patches. Their efficacy appears good and some reports of reduced side-effects support their use. However, the long time to reach steady state and limited dose options makes titration difficult and prolonged. Knowledge of equivalent morphine dose and patch pharmacokinetics is essential to obtain optimal safe analgesia if patches are to be considered.

Drugs should be prescribed by one doctor and issued from one pharmacy.

10.7 Tolerance, dependence and drug addiction

Tolerance is reduced responsiveness to the effects of a drug caused by its previous administration with increasing the dose required to produce the same effect previously produced by a smaller dose. In chronic pain, once a stable dose has been achieved tolerance is seldom a problem. However, there is an initial dose titration phase, which can take weeks. Patients requesting higher doses during this phase should not be treated with suspicion.

Dependence is characterized by a compulsion to take the drug in order to experience its physical effects and avoid the discomfort of its absence. Psychological dependence is a compulsion to take the drug because of the need for stimulation, or because it relieves anxiety or depression. Physical dependence is characterized by an intense physical disturbance when the drug is withdrawn. **Patients who successfully use opioids for pain relief may be physically dependent upon them although very few will be psychologically dependent.**

Addiction is a cluster of behavioural, cognitive and psychological phenomena that develop after repeated substance use. There is a strong desire to take the drug, difficulties in controlling its use despite harmful consequences and a higher priority given to drug use than to other activities and obligations. It is rare for patients with chronic pain to develop an addiction but when it does occur it can cause severe mental and physical problems with resultant difficulties for carers and medical staff. Careful patient selection and monitoring are essential and, if problems occur, prompt involvement of secondary care services such as multidisciplinary pain management clinics and addiction services prove invaluable.

Behaviours that should prompt concern

- earlier prescription seeking; claims of lost medication
- unsanctioned dose escalation
- requesting specific drugs
- acquiring drugs from other medical sources
- evidence of intoxication
- missed appointments
- coexistent use of illicit drugs
- use of drug to treat other symptoms

10.8 What about follow-up?

At the one week monitoring visit, Danielle reported significant pain relief although she felt drowsy and nauseous. Her sleep had improved but her husband said she slept a lot of the day and was concerned. As a result, her functional level had not improved.

The dose of MST was reduced to 10mg twice daily and she was again encouraged to become more active during the day. A simple goal of walking down the road twice a day was agreed.

Regular patient monitoring is essential, particularly during the titration phase. Monitoring visits should focus on analgesia, the presence of side-effects and their management, and the evaluation of functional goals.

At subsequent follow-up visits Danielle reported that the nausea and drowsiness had significantly improved, thus enabling a progressive increase to a dose of 30mg MST twice daily over the next three months. Once analgesia was established, functional assessments and physiotherapy achieved a significant improvement.

10.9 Summary

There is growing evidence that some patients with chronic non-malignant pain may benefit from the use of long-term oral strong opioids. The challenge facing medical carers is alleviating the suffering without increasing illicit use, addiction, or medication-induced suffering. Whereas the evidence for the use of opioids for nociceptive chronic pain is clear, the use of opioids in neuropathic pain is more contentious; the role of the pain team can play an important role in the decision to use opioids.

Choosing appropriate patients, using the correct drug as part of a multidisciplinary plan and regular assessment of progress and problems should enable strong opioids to be of value in patients who may have few other options.

Bibliography

Allen, L. and Hayes, H. Randomised crossover trial of transdermal fentanyl and sustained release morphine for treating chronic non-cancer pain. *Br. Med. J.*, **322**, 1154.

Anon. (2004). Recommendations for the appropriate use of opioids for persistent non-cancer pain. The Pain Society (in collaboration with the Royal College of Anaesthetists, the Royal College of General Practitioners and the Royal College of Psychatrists), March 2004.

Breivik, H. Opioids in cancer and chronic non-cancer pain therapy—indications and controversies. *Acta Anaesth. Scand.*, **45**, 1059–1066.

Collett, B.J. Opioid tolerance: the clinical perspective. *Br. J. Anaesth.*, **81**, 58–68.

McQuay, H. (1999). Pain: opioids in pain management. *Lancet*, **353**, 2229–2232.

Chapter 11

Pain of urological and genital origin

Andrew Baranowski

The following chapter covers pain of urological and genital origin. It serves as an example of how more complex pains may be approached employing a team effort. The chapter also illustrates how pain medicine is developing and how an understanding of anatomy and physiology may help in the understanding of presenting symptoms and signs.

Chronic pelvic pain (CPP) is a term that is used to describe chronic pain that appears to stem from within the organs of the pelvis. It may arise as a result of pathology within the pelvis but may also arise from structures outside e.g. the nervous system or referred from the spine. As a consequence, assessments of CPP must include these systems. Due to common mechanisms, vulval pain and pain perceived in the external male genitalia are considered to fall within the definition of pelvic pain.

11.1 David's perineal pain

David, a very distressed 34-year-old, was referred to the pain clinic by his GP with six months of vague, non-specific pain in the perineum. It radiated to his penis and testicles and was aggravated by sitting and urination. He put up with the pain for a few weeks because a similar pain a few years ago had resolved. Now he felt that this latest pain was becoming worse. There were times when he found his legs were stiff and did not appear to work properly; he often felt nauseous and quite 'ill'. He was sure he had 'spikes of temperature'. However, there was no history consistent with haematuria or puss in the urine. Urination was difficult to start, with a poor and interrupted flow. He had lost interest in sex with weak erections and painful ejaculation.

Investigations by his GP and then urologists showed no signs of infection and David was consistently apyrexial. Repeated clinical examinations, which included neurological and rectal, were normal along with routine blood tests and a transrectal ultrasound of the pelvis. Despite this David had been given several courses of antibiotics. He had also been prescribed simple analgesics.

The priority of those initially assessing David was to ensure that he was not suffering from an acute infection or any other serious pathology such as a tumour. The history could easily have been consistent with these. Whereas cystitis in a man is uncommon, it may occur; it can be ruled out by simple urine dipstick tests and urinary culture. Most patients will not have positive urine cultures, but many will still be labelled with the diagnosis of 'prostatitis'. In most cases the term 'prostatitis' is a misnomer, as patients rarely have an infected or even inflamed prostate.

To further investigate the possible diagnosis of 'prostatitis', David went on to have a prostatic massage and cystoscopy. The massage was aimed at collecting prostatic secretions for microscopy and culture: the Stamey test. The prostatic massage was painful for David but afterwards he had less pain. No inflammatory cells were identified and similarly microbial culture was negative. On cystoscopy, his bladder was slightly inflamed and a diagnosis of interstitial cystitis was suggested.

In the absence of proven inflammation or infection of the prostate it is difficult to be sure that the pain is coming from the prostate. It has been suggested that infection may be loculated within the prostate, but this theory has little support. In the absence of proven infection, only two courses of broad-spectrum, prostate-penetrating antibiotics should be considered. The exact antibiotics will vary from practice to practice.

David found the rectal examination and massage painful but this does not necessarily mean that the pain is originating from the prostate. Tenderness of the prostatic area has to be clearly differentiated from tenderness of other structures such as the pelvic floor muscles or the pudendal nerve. Modern pelvic pain terminology aims to reflect this (see Box 11.1). It has been suggested that benefit following prostatic massage may be due to the coincidental stretching of pelvic floor muscles. Dysfunction of the pelvic floor muscles may also be the cause of the urinary symptoms that David suffers with. Spasm of these muscles may lead to urinary frequency, urgency, hesitancy and poor flow—all the urinary symptoms that David was complaining of.

During cystoscopy, even if no infection is proven, the bladder wall may look inflamed as it did in David's case. If the bladder is extremely inflamed the diagnosis of interstitial cystitis (IC) needs to be considered. IC is a very specific term based upon specific research criteria; it is only one of the many painful bladder syndromes. The cause of IC is poorly understood; it is suggested that the bladder becomes inflamed as a result of a neurogenic process similar to a complex regional pain syndrome (see elsewhere in this book). As a consequence, inflammatory-type changes of the bladder do not necessarily indicate that the primary pathology is in the bladder.

Box 11.1 Extract from the European Association of Urology Guidelines on Chronic Pelvic Pain, 2002

Definitions extracted from the *European Association of Urology Guidelines on Chronic Pelvic Pain (CCP)*. Urogenital pain syndromes are a collection of symptoms and signs where the aetiology is often poorly understood.

- *Chronic pelvic pain* is non-malignant pain perceived in structures related to the pelvis in men or women. In nociceptive pain that becomes chronic, the pain must have been continuous or recurrent for at least six months. If non-acute pain mechanisms are documented then the pain may be regarded as chronic irrespective of the time period. In all cases, there may be associated cognitive, behavioural and social consequences. Well defined conditions producing chronic pain, as well as pain syndromes, are included in this definition.

Examples of pain syndromes: In the absence of proven infection or other obvious pathology–

- *Pelvic pain syndrome* is the occurrence of persistent or recurrent episodic pelvic pain associated with symptoms suggestive of lower urinary tract, sexual, bowel or gynaecological dysfunction.
- *Bladder pain syndrome* is suprapubic pain related to bladder filling, accompanied by other symptoms such as increased urinary frequency.
- *Prostate pain syndrome* is the occurrence of persistent or recurrent episodic prostate pain, which is associated with symptoms suggestive of urinary tract and/or sexual dysfunction.
- *Pelvic floor muscle pain syndrome* is the occurrence of persistent or recurrent, episodic, pelvic floor pain with associated trigger-points that is either related to the micturition cycle or associated with symptoms suggestive of urinary tract or sexual dysfunction.
- *Pudendal pain syndrome* is a neuropathic-type pain arising in the distribution of the pudendal nerve with symptoms and signs of rectal, urinary tract or sexual dysfunction.

David was seen by a specialist urologist and it was decided that he did not meet the research criteria for IC and the diagnosis of bladder pain syndrome was suggested. As it was felt that David did not have a well-defined urological problem he was referred to the pain clinic. At the initial consultation with the pain clinic, David met an environment very different from the acute and hectic urology clinic. A more general history was undertaken.

David was a high flying businessman, with a wife and two young children. He was physically active, and enjoyed sports which included cycling. During his life he had suffered a number of sports injuries, which included a groin strain whilst playing football and a 'slipped disc' at the gym. With his work he spent a lot of time travelling and it was apparent that he had not always been faithful to his wife. Work was stressful with David having to meet many deadlines. He admitted to anxiety and to being depressed.

The history is a very important part of the pain assessment. Occasionally traumatic life experiences may be relevant (Box 11.2). The interaction may be complicated and often requires the skills of an experienced pain management psychologist to separate out the issues that are relevant to an individual's pain. In a number of cases the pain may occur as a psychological response to the key life event (possibly a psychosomatic response)—such a response is considered to be rare and the link has even been disputed. In many cases the pain is a constant reminder of the distressing event (a post-traumatic stress response type of response). Probably, all patients with CPP will suffer psychological consequences as a result of their pain and its associated disability. There will be specific psychosexual issues in the case of most patients with CPP and these may require specific interventions with a pain management psychologist.

In David's case, the relationship with his wife and family needs to be considered and the consultant in pain medicine felt that the skills of a pain psychologist were necessary. The consultant was aware that psychological issues might be secondary to the pain and not the primary factor. The significance of the adultery was also not clear. However, the main reason for referring to a pain management psychologist was so that David could look at his coping strategies and explore a cognitive–behavioural approach to pain management.

Box 11.2 Traumatic life events that may be associated with CPP

- history of trauma
  - sexual abuse
  - rape
  - torture
- negative awareness of sexuality experience
  - traumatic menarche
  - traumatic first sexual experience
  - traumatic homosexual awakening
- tragic loss
  - death of partner
  - divorce
  - adultery
  - loss of employment

Association of CPP with a traumatic life event does not necessarily mean that the life event is the cause of pain, but the pain may act as a reminder.

David had begun to recognize that stress was making his pain worse and this was certainly an area that David could work on with the psychologist.

During David's initial assessment at the pain clinic, a further thorough examination was undertaken. No evidence of the old 'slipped disc' could be found and the consultant was satisfied that the pain did not stem from the back. Examinations of the entheses (tendon attachments) in the region of the groin were tender but did not reproduce David's pain. Rectal examination demonstrated trigger points within the pelvic floor muscles. There was minimal tenderness in the region of the prostate or over the course of the pudendal nerves. There was no perineal or penile numbness; the bulbocavernosus reflex was intact.

The consultant had ruled out spinal pathology as a cause of the pain and so no further investigations of the spine were indicated. There was no overt evidence of pudendal nerve damage, so specific scans of the course of the pudendal nerve and nerve conduction tests were not indicated. Diagnostic blocks of the pudendal nerve could be considered, as these are sometimes helpful even in the absence of overt pudendal neurology. Such injections may assist management in patients with pelvic floor muscle spasm or central sensitization.

The consultant in pain medicine spent a lot of time explaining to David that he had been fully investigated and that no serious pathology had been found. A model of pain involving muscle dysfunction was explained. The role of the central nervous system in maintaining the pain as well as in sensitising the bladder was also discusssed. It was explained that the whole system can be stirred up by the psychological response to stress. A trial of transcutaneous electrical nerve stimulation (TENS) was also suggested and an electromyographic (EMG) study of the pelvic floor muscles. David's pelvic muscles were demonstrated to be hyperactive and he was taught how to train the muscles using biofeedback. A specialist practitioner also performed a release of pelvic floor muscle trigger points.

In the absence of specific pathology, the model described above (reassurance, pain management psychology, pelvic floor education and simple pain management techniques such as TENS) can produce significant benefit and is often more rewarding than surgery. Adjuvant analgesics such as antidepressants and anticonvulsants may also have a role.

David occasionally had setbacks and it took many months, but he did make steady progress. The pain reduced progressively but more significantly there was a reduction in his disability and psychological distress. Constant reassurance was necessary and appropriate.

11.2 **Summary points for chronic pelvic pain**

- The physical assessment should be comprehensive and include the neuromuscular system outside of the pelvis.
- Physical interventions may be therapeutic but often also have an important diagnostic role.
- Neuropathic adjuvant drugs may reduce symptoms.
- In the absence of specific physical pathology, a detailed psychological assessment will form the cornerstone of further management.
- Even in the presence of ongoing physical pathology, a cognitive behavioural approach to the disease and pain management may reduce pain, disability and psychological distress.

Bibliography

Egan K.J. and Krieger, J.L. (1997). Chronic abacterial prostatitis—a urological chronic pain syndrome? *Pain,* **69**, 213–218.

Fall, M. and Lindstrom, S. (1994). Transcutaneous electrical nerve stimulation in classic and nonulcer interstitial cystitis. *Urol. Clin. North. Am.* **21**, 131–139.

Fall, M. (chair), Baranowski, A.P., Fowler, C.J., Lepinard, V., Malone-Lee, J.G., Messelink, E.J., Oberpenning, F., Osborne, J.L., and Schumacher. S.(2004). Guidelines on chronic pelvic pain. *Eur. Urol.*, **46**, 681–689.

Howard, F.M. (2000). Pelvic floor pain syndrome. In: Howard, F.M., ed. *Pelvic Pain. Diagnosis and Management,* pp. 429–432. Lippincott/ Williams & Wilkins, Philadelphia.

Wenninger, K., Heiman, J.R., Rothman, I., Berghuis, J.P., and Berger, R.E. (1996). Sickness impact of chronic nonbacterial prostatitis and its correlates. *J. Urol.* **155**, 965–968.

Chapter 12

Cancer pain

James de Courcy

Pain is common in cancer but not universal. It affects up to 70% of patients. The good news is that despite these initially discouraging statistics, relatively simple approaches can manage the majority of patients' pain effectively. These approaches have many features in common with many outlined elsewhere in this volume, and to avoid duplication in this brief overview detailed discussion of the various pain types, drug groups and treatments will not be repeated here.

12.1 Marie's cancer and her pain

A 38-year-old married nurse with two young children was referred to the Pain Management Service with aching pain in her left anterior thigh, some weakness of the quadriceps muscles, and a burning, aching, tender pain in the right shoulder. A year previously, Marie had received radiotherapy following a hysterectomy for cervical carcinoma. On examination there was minimal dullness to pinprick and light touch in her femoral nerve distribution, and tenderness in the femoral triangle. Imaging revealed recurrent tumour with some cystic change invading down the femoral canal with compression of the femoral nerve. Examination of the shoulder revealed a palpable tender, myofascial trigger point in the belly of the trapezius muscle, and pressure over this reproduced her shoulder pain.

At the time of presentation she was receiving regular co-proxamol which was not controlling her pain. This was converted to regular immediate-release oral morphine administered four-hourly with breakthrough doses available, supplemented with regular naproxen and, because of the compression of the femoral nerve, introduction of a small dose of dexamethasone. In addition, fluid was drained from the cystic part of the tumour under ultrasound guidance. She was referred to the oncologist for consideration of radiotherapy to the tumour since this lay outside the previously treated field. Reassurance about its benign nature and subsequent use of a transcutaneous electrical nerve stimulation (TENS) machine proved effective for the shoulder pain. In order to prevent opioid-induced constipation she was commenced on a combined stimulant and softener laxative before she developed these symptoms.

Following the above, Marie gained good control of the pain and was able to be discharged home for a number of weeks. Unfortunately her pain then rapidly worsened and became uncontrolled. Assessment revealed further weakness of the quadriceps, with spontaneous shooting pains and pain with light touch (allodynia) in the femoral nerve distribution. A diagnosis of neuropathic pain due to invasion of the femoral nerve by the tumour was made. Addition of amitriptyline and subsequently gabapentin to the morphine and dexamethasone gave partial relief and this was further improved with the addition of mexiletine (a local anaesthetic drug available for oral use, normally used to treat cardiac conduction disturbances and occasionally helpful in neuropathic pain).

Unfortunately, after a short period of improved relief, the pain control worsened again with severe neuropathic pain in the leg. After discussion with the patient, her family and the primary care team, a tunnelled percutaneous intrathecal catheter was sited at L2/3 and a continuous infusion of bupivacaine, a local anaesthetic, and diamorphine was commenced via a portable battery-powered pump. Excellent pain control was rapidly gained, and after education of the community nursing team on management of the catheter and pump she was discharged home, with routine care of the catheter and infusion being delivered by the community nurses with support and regular follow-up by the pain management team. On this regime she remained comfortable at home for some months until her death.

12.2 Treat the whole patient

This case illustrates some important principles in cancer pain management. Assessment of patients with cancer pain should take a very holistic approach. For many patients, the return of pain implies a recurrence of their cancer and impending death which leads to concern about the family and the future. This anxiety will greatly worsen their overall experience and ability to cope with the pain: this has been described by Saunders as 'Total Pain'. In addition, sleep patterns and other symptoms not directly related to pain (e.g. constipation, nausea and fatigue) should all be addressed. All professionals involved should address the wider psychological and social aspects as well. Understanding that assessment may be difficult because of the reluctance of many patients to complain of pain may mean that probing and direct questions are necessary. As illustrated by this case, most patients experience multiple pains from different causes with different mechanisms. Not all of these may respond well to opioids and for this reason adjuvant drugs may be required. Again, like Marie's shoulder pain, not all the sources of pain are malignant and assessment of this with reassurance can be invaluable.

12.3 Pharmacotherapy

The mainstay of pharmacotherapy is the use of oral opioids, principally morphine, though other alternatives may sometimes be of use. The World Health Organization (WHO) ladder of analgesia and the principles underlying the use of these drugs are now well known.

Opioids in cancer pain—key points

- by the mouth, by the clock, by the ladder and individualized for the patient
- use of the WHO analgesic ladder with adjuvant treatments
- dosage titration: regular four-hourly administration; titrate up dose in adequate increments: 30–50% increase every two days
- adequate breakthrough dose size:1/6 of the total daily dose
- once a stable effective dose is established, convert to sustained release preparation with an immediate-release breakthrough dose
- a combination of stimulant and softener laxatives should be prescribed automatically—constipation is a very common and troublesome, easier prevented than treated
- anti-emetics should be prescribed if necessary but nausea is not universal and tends to diminish after a few days
- morphine is the principal drug, but other drugs may have advantages

However, some pains may not respond well to opioids, and for these, other drug groups may be used. Such pains may be divided into opioid 'partially responsive' and 'poorly responsive', the former responding to an opioid in conjunction with an adjuvant drug such a steroid (e.g. the nerve compression pain above), or non-steroidal anti-inflammatory drugs in pains such as those from bony metastases.

Neuropathic pain is one of those that is common in cancer patients and typically not responsive to opioids; it may occur from nerve invasion or spinal metastases. For this, tricyclic antidepressants, anticonvulsants, membrane-stabilizing drugs such as mexiletine or lignocaine, or n-methyl d-aspartate (NMDA) receptor antagonists such as ketamine or amantadine are all options. The latter two categories (membrane stabilizers and NMDA receptor antagonists) would normally be initiated by a specialist team. A neuropathic pain ladder analogous to the WHO opioid ladder approach has been described (see Table 12.1).

Figure 12.1 Neuropathic pain ladder for cancer pain patients

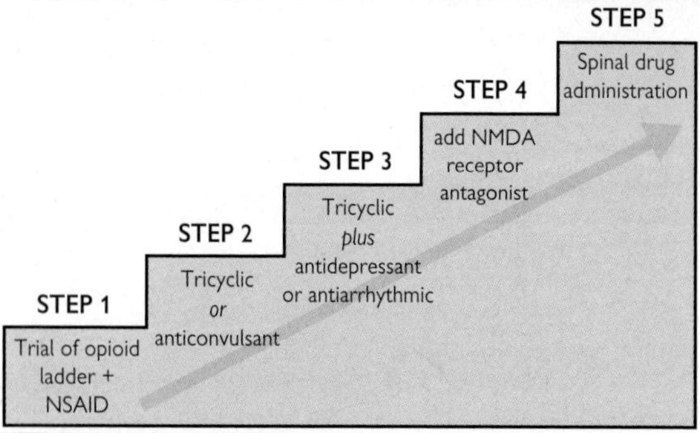

Table 12.1 Treatment approaches of different pain types

Pain type	Likely opioid response	Treatment options
Visceral and soft tissue	Good	Opioid ladder ± adjuvants
Bone	Partial	Opioid ladder + NSAID
Nerve compression	Partial	Opioid ladder + steroid
Nerve destruction	Poor	Tricyclic antidepressants, anticonvulsants, mexiletine and ketamine
Myofascial	Poor	Tricyclic antidepressants, TENS, acupuncture
Spasticity	Poor	Muscle relaxants
Visceral spasm	Poor	Antispasmodics

12.4 **Physical methods**

As well as pharmacological approaches, the use of physical methods such as TENS may aid pain control and additionally have the psychological advantage of being something that patients themselves can use for self-management. Acupuncture and massage may give relief particularly in myofascial pain and spasm, which is very common in cancer patients.

Neuropathic pain in cancer

Common symptoms:

- allodynia—what should be felt as light touch is painful
- hyperalgesia—exaggerated response to a normally painful stimulus
- dysaesthesia—unpleasant abnormal sensation, spontaneous or provoked
- hyperpathia—abnormally painful reaction to a stimulus, especially repetitive, with increased threshold and often prolonged duration
- anaesthesia dolorosa—pain in an area of numbness

Drug classes:

- antidepressants: for most pains, first line, e.g. amitriptyline
- anticonvulsants, e.g. sodium valproate, gabapentin, pregabalin
- antiarrhythmics, e.g. mexiletine
- NMDA receptor antagonists, e.g. ketamine, amantadine

12.5 Other treatments and spinal drugs

With many types of pain such as that from bony metastases and others such as the nerve compression in Marie's case, one should consider whether there is a place for radiotherapy, chemotherapy or surgical decompression or stabilization of, for example, an incipient fracture.

Nerve block techniques can sometimes be used to provide pain relief. They may be temporary with local anaesthetic with or without depot steroids; destructive using chemical agents (e.g. phenol or alcohol); or physical methods (e.g. radiofrequency lesioning and cryotherapy). With the exception of coeliac plexus blocks for upper abdominal malignancy, destructive nerve block techniques have become less common with increased use of spinal drug administration. Nevertheless, the effects of local anaesthetic blocks can sometimes last for a usefully long period, particularly when combined with a depot steroid preparation.

In a very few cases where, as in this case, all other methods of analgesia have proved inadequate, delivery of opioids and other drugs directly to the spinal cord where they act may prove necessary: the commonest indication is failure to obtain adequate analgesia by oral routes due to excessive side-effects. Both intrathecal (with a catheter within the cerebrospinal fluid) and epidural (with a catheter just outside the dura) techniques are used. It is most useful to use a combination of local anaesthetic and opioid with or without other drugs such as clonidine as these are synergistic and offer the chance of excellent analgesia with minimal side-effects. Neurogenic pain may respond well to local anaesthetics. Various studies have looked at the cost-effectiveness and results of tunnelled percutaneous catheters against totally implanted pumps, and the former compare well for most of these patients with limited life expectancy.

12.6 Where should patients be managed?

With the well-recognized desire of the majority of patients to remain at home at the end of their life, the full involvement of the primary care team in the management of pain is vital, and as in this case even 'high-tech' invasive techniques can be managed safely in the community with the support of the specialist pain management team. However, it is relatively unusual to have to resort to this sort of management and effective application of simple measures such as the analgesic ladder, with appropriate use of adjuvant techniques, will result in effective management of the pain in most patients with cancer.

12.7 Summary points

- Careful assessment is of paramount importance.
- Tailoring of treatment to likely source of the pain.
- Multiple sources and types of pain.
- Multimodal approach.
- Analgesic ladder with adjuvants.
- Consider radiotherapy and surgery.
- Other drugs.
- Nerve blocks and infusions.

Bibliography

Back,I.N. *Palliative Medicine Handbook*. http://book.pallcare.info/index.php (with permission from Dr Back).

Expert working group of the European Association for Palliative Care (2001). Morphine and alternative opioids in cancer pain: the EAPC guidelines. *Br. J. Cancer* **84**, 587–593 or http://www.eapcnet.org/publications/research.asp.

Regnard, C.F.B. and Tempest, S. (1998). *A guide to Symptom Relief in Advanced Disease* (4th edn). Hochland & Hochland.

Twycross, R.G. (1994). *Pain Relief in Advanced Cancer*. Churchill Livingstone, Edinburgh.

Twycross, R. and Wilcock, A. (2001). *Symptom Management in Advanced Cancer*. Radcliffe Medical Press, Abingdon.

Chapter 13

Psychological aspects of pain

Anna Mandeville and Kate Ridout

Cognitive behavioural therapy (CBT) is increasingly recognised as an intrinsically appropriate aspect of the treatment of many long-term medical problems. There is a strong evidence base for its use in reducing disability and distress in the context of chronic pain. A CBT approach to pain is often delivered via an in- or outpatient group pain management program, usually led by a clinical psychologist and supported by other disciplines. This chapter provides an introduction to the key ways in which CBT can be used in the treatment of someone with pain.

A key component in the experience of pain is a person's cognitive response. This refers to the person's thoughts and feelings about the meaning of the pain and their expectations in relation to it. For example, in response to acute pain a person may have the thought and expectation 'this pain will be better in a few days'. They may then rest a while, getting back to normal activity levels as the pain subsides. However, if pain persists, anxiety can develop as more negative predictions about the pain and its impact are made. For example, thoughts like 'by the end of the day I'll be in agony—I will have to rest in bed', or 'last time I tried to do any exercise I was much worse, so it must be dangerous to move' may lead to a reduction in activity and a fear of re-injury. Depression, disability and physical deconditioning can then follow as a chronic pain syndrome develops.

CBT helps a person to evaluate and challenge thoughts they have about their pain. It is assumed that many thoughts about pain are in fact distortions which overestimate the threat that the pain poses. For example, a person may be able to challenge the thought that their pain is so excessive that they have to spend the day in bed resting. This would involve a re-evaluation, such as 'even though my pain feels worse today, if I pace myself carefully taking frequent breaks and do an extra relaxation session I may still be able to achieve some of the tasks I planned'. These modified thoughts are much more likely to produce increased activity and encourage the re-development of confidence and stamina.

CBT and chronic pain

- thoughts about pain lead to patterns of feelings and behaviours
- thoughts about pain are coloured by anxiety and become distorted
- distorted thoughts, e.g. about the risk of re-injury, lead the person to engage in unhelpful behaviours, e.g. reducing activity
- reducing activity leads to low mood, physical deconditioning and preoccupation with pain
- CBT can help a person to challenge unhelpful thoughts and substitute more useful ones which lead to more adaptive behaviour

If this can be done early enough in the course of a person's experience of pain, it may then play a role in preventing the development of chronic pain. The following case example illustrates the application of a cognitive approach in more detail.

13.1 **Nick has neck pain**

Nick is a 39-year-old father of four. He works as a street market trader and is married to Jan, a secretary. Nick began to experience pain in his neck and jaw about two years prior to referral. The onset of the pain was gradual and Nick himself associates it with a very busy period at work when he spent a lot of time moving stock from storage to the markets and long hours doing his book keeping. Initially Nick increased his use of 'over-the-counter' analgesics and maintained his work pattern. However, when the pain did not remit, he sought treatment from his GP who prescribed him co-codamol and referred him to the rheumatology department at his local hospital and for physiotherapy. Various blood tests and imaging failed to pinpoint clearly the aetiology of the pain. Although physiotherapy initially helped, his pain persisted.

Nick began to be more worried about his pain. In particular, he began to worry that lifting stock at work may be making his pain worse. Gradually, he asked his assistants to do more and more of the heavy lifting as he became increasingly anxious about his pain. Nick had previously enjoyed playing football, but began to avoid this as he worried that he might injure himself further and make the pain worse. He began to spend more time thinking about the pain, fearing that something 'serious' was going on and that the doctors had 'missed something'. He started to avoid going out as he became increasingly worried that his pain 'might get on top of him', especially in social situations. This was associated with fears that he might embarrass himself and his wife if the pain became severe and he had to make excuses to others in order to return home. He also began

Nick's cognitions and pain behaviour

- Nick increasingly avoids physical activity through fear of making the pain worse
- Nick has more anxious thoughts about disease which may underlie his pain
- Nick begins to avoid social situations through fear of embarrassment
- Thoughts about not being a 'good father' drive Nick to 'overdo' activities and cause flare-ups in his pain
- Nick's mood deteriorates and his business is affected

to withdraw from involvement in family life. Occasionally he would feel guilty about the fact that he was less able to play football with his sons and 'force himself' to play with them for a whole afternoon. The next day he invariably found his pain was worse and this increased his belief that it was better to avoid exercise altogether. Nick's business began to suffer as his confidence decreased and he became more and more withdrawn.

13.2 CBT intervention

There were many opportunities to intervene cognitively in Nick's case. Educating Nick about the benefits of sustaining movement and teaching him ways of mobilizing and lifting safely had the potential to help him decrease his fear of exacerbating the pain and hence maintain activity. Helping him to incorporate new information could result in his generating more helpful patterns of thinking for himself. Examples of this might be: 'I may need to ask people to help me to lift very heavy loads at the moment but this is short term. If I pace my lifting with regular breaks and stretching to relieve muscle tension, I will gradually be able to increase getting back to lifting myself, without worrying too much about injuring myself further.'

Nick's fears about having something 'seriously wrong' can also be confronted using a cognitive approach. For example, thoughts such as 'the doctors have missed something and later they will find out I have a progressive disease like multiple sclerosis' can be challenged. This involves collaborating with the person in weighing up the evidence and likelihood of this possibility and exploring whether symptoms could be attributed to benign causes such as muscle tension. Nick could also be encouraged to weigh up the consequences of thinking catastrophically (i.e. the outcome will be the worst possible scenario). The emphasis here is on exploring the possibility that other explanations might be equally likely, not on totally arguing against the original anxious thoughts.

CBT intervention

- tackling Nick's fear of further injury
  - challenging and replacing his distorted thoughts
  - providing education about mobilizing safely
  - helping Nick to gradually increase activity levels under supervision
- helping Nick to re-estimate the likelihood of serious underlying illness
- teaching Nick to manage his thoughts and behaviours in social situations in a more helpful way
- helping Nick to see that being a 'good father' can be achieved without putting himself at risk of a major flare-up

Nick could be helped to challenge his thoughts about avoiding social activities. He might be encouraged to build up his social life again gradually, starting with shorter trips out. This could be done whilst helping Nick to challenge thoughts such as 'this pain is unbearable and I have to go home' and replace them with self-statements such as 'although I am aware of the pain I know that going home will not really make much difference; it may help me to feel less anxious, but I know that if I stay in this situation and do my breathing exercises slowly, I can get through the next twenty minutes and I will review the situation then'.

Finally, Nick could be helped to explore and challenge thoughts involving guilt and fear about not being involved enough with his sons. These anxious thoughts had previously led Nick to 'overdo' activity, with a resultant flare-up of pain, thus confirming his beliefs that all activity leads to increased pain. Exploring his thinking about fatherhood might help him to recognize that there are many ways of being a 'good father' that don't involve excessive 'overdoing' of activity.

This kind of CBT intervention contributes towards decreasing Nick's disability and distress in relation to pain, as he builds confidence in returning to pleasurable activities, despite pain. If left untreated, fear and avoidance of activity are typical factors which may contribute to acute pain becoming increasingly chronic. Individuals' beliefs about pain can be frightening for patients and quite strongly held. Therefore, intervening cognitively demands patience on the part of therapists as they assist an individual in gradually testing out and modifying their anxious thoughts and fears.

Pain management programmes (see also Chapter 14)

- this is a specific phrase which means a group based programme working with cognitive-behavioural techniques
- the groups are usually led by a clinical psychologist supported by a specialist physiotherapist; they may also be assisted by a doctor, a nurse or an occupational therapist
- they run over several weeks as inpatient or outpatient programmes, and are usually subject to regular audit of outcomes
- these programs aim to reduce the disability and distress associated with chronic pain
- the British Pain Society has recently produced guidelines for high quality pain management programmes

Bibliography

Erskine, A. and Williams, A.C., de C. (1989). Chronic pain. In: Broome, A. (ed.) *Health Psychology, Processes and Applications.* Chapman & Hall, London.

Morley. S., Eccleston, C., Williams, A.C., de C. (1999). Systematic review and meta-analysis of randomised controlled trials of cognitive behaviour therapy and behaviour therapy for chronic pain in adults, excluding headache. *Pain*, **80**, 1–13.

Chapter 14

Non-medical treatment in managing people with long-term pain

Kelly Wynne

Chronic musculoskeletal pain is a common and benign problem, yet it can have an enormous effect on an individual's quality of life and ability to work. One in five people in the UK receive incapacity benefits because of chronic musculoskeletal pain, representing a considerable economic burden to society. In this chapter, the role of non-medical approaches will be discussed in treating people with long-term pain. The emphasis on management is not only to relieve pain, but also to reduce disability.

14.1 Pain relief

When patients develop chronic pain, the question most will have for their GP is 'Is there a cure?' There are a number of pain-relieving treatments available for patients with chronic musculoskeletal pain. The following treatments are offered in most pain clinics in the UK and could be offered to the patient in primary care. Having some of these treatments available to patients in a primary care setting could help to ensure fast and easy access to successful pain treatments without a referral to a pain clinic.

14.2 Transcutaneous electrical nerve stimulation (TENS)

TENS machines are cheap, easy to use and have almost no side-effects. They can provide 'drug-free pain relief' for some patients. The evidence base for the use of TENS in the treatment of chronic musculoskeletal pain is inconclusive. Further information regarding the evidence for the use of TENS in chronic musculoskeletal pain is available on the Cochrane Library web site.

14.3 Acupuncture and trigger-point injections

Acupuncture can be performed according to Eastern or Western principles. Trigger-point injections involve injecting a local anaesthetic into a trigger point (areas of muscle that have become tight and tender to touch). The exact pathophysiology of trigger points is unknown. The evidence base for the use of acupuncture in chronic musculoskeletal pain is inconclusive. More research is also needed to determine the efficacy of trigger-point injections in the treatment of chronic musculoskeletal pain.

All pain-relieving treatments for chronic musculoskeletal pain need to be closely monitored and evaluated against meaningful functional outcomes. Long-term pain relief alongside sustained improvements in function and return to work must be demonstrated if the practitioner is to be sure that the treatment is really of benefit. If the patient is 'feeling better' following treatment but remains unable to get back to work or normal activity other treatments or an immediate referral to a pain clinic should be considered.

14.4 Pain management

Some patients can be cured or gain substantial relief from pain-relieving treatments. However, there are a small number of patients who become increasingly distressed and disabled by chronic musculoskeletal pain. Their management often poses a considerable challenge to the practitioner. These patients can often consume large amounts of healthcare and welfare resources. It is widely accepted that beliefs and attitudes regarding chronic pain and not the pain itself determine whether or not a patient becomes severely disabled. Unhelpful beliefs need to be understood and corrected in primary care if the patient has any chance of staying employed and active.

Here are our Top 5 Pain Management Tips for reducing disability and distress in the patient with chronic musculoskeletal pain.

1. Do not re-investigate chronic musculoskeletal pain unless you feel it is absolutely necessary; it can reinforce a patient's fear that something is seriously wrong and increase psychological distress.
2. Correct unhelpful beliefs about chronic musculoskeletal pain; terms such as 'degeneration' and 'trapped nerves' can promote fear of injury and disability.
3. Explain that 'pain does not mean damage' in chronic benign musculoskeletal pain.
4. Explain how chronic pain is different from acute pain and educate the family if they are also distressed.
5. If concerned that the patient is becoming increasingly disabled despite interventions, refer them to a pain clinic sooner rather than later.

14.5 Pain management programmes

When pain-relieving treatments available in pain clinics and elsewhere prove unsuccessful and chronic pain continues to cause considerable disability and suffering, referral to a pain management programme should be considered. Pain management programmes utilize cognitive behavioural strategies to enable individuals with chronic pain to reduce the impact that the pain is having on their lives. Pain management programmes help patients with chronic pain to regain control over the lives by teaching them psychological strategies and increasing their levels of activity and fitness. There is evidence that pain management programmes significantly reduce psychological distress and disability in patients with chronic musculoskeletal pain. Pain management programmes run across the country either as inpatient residential programmes or on an outpatient basis. There are also residential pain management programmes for adolescents with chronic pain and disability, for instance in Bath, UK. Many programmes will accept primary care referrals from across the UK.

Patients that have sometimes been signed off work and who are generally distressed and overwhelmed by their pain can assume the worst about the severity of their problem. Here are some examples of the management of chronic musculoskeletal pain in primary care, which actually reduced the impact of chronic pain on the lives of patients and their families.

14.6 Simple back pain managed by a GP

James, a 45-year-old store manager developed severe low back pain without any radiation to the leg following some do-it-yourself at home. He was physically supported into the clinic by his partner. The patient stated that he was worried that he might have 'slipped a disc' and caused some serious damage. After some discussion it became clear that James had been having increasingly frequent attacks of low back pain over the last seven months and that currently he had back pain most of the time. To manage the increases in pain James had stopped attending the gym and lifting heavy objects at home or work, and was trying to rest in bed during the weekends. He had also seen a physiotherapist and a chiropractor privately, but this had not stopped the attacks. In fact, this had been the worst attack yet. After ruling out the possibility of serious pathology, the GP diagnosed recurrent simple low back pain, prescribed some non-steroidal anti-inflammatory drugs and reassured James that although the back pain was intense it should resolve over time. Clear advice was given on staying active to promote recovery and James was given a copy of *The Back Book*. Recurrence was discussed openly as very likely and the patient was invited to think about how he could cope with future episodes of back pain and how stamina, strength and suppleness was essential in this condition. The primary care doctor and James discussed how he might manage work with increased low back pain, by taking regular breaks through the day and performing difficult work tasks 'little and often'. Some of the discussion took place with the partner present, to calm her fears about what was happening and to allow her to reinforce helpful behaviour like exercise and return to work. James was urged to start lifting again, to strengthen the back but to build up slowly.

Six months later James saw the primary care doctor for an unrelated problem and commented that he was lifting at work, was attending the gym and his attacks of low back pain had reduced in frequency and severity. He remarked that his partner had been especially good as she had taken the kids to allow him to attend the gym and reminded him how important it was to go regularly, especially if his back was sore.

14.7 Managing a patient with 15 years of pain

Anusha, a 55-year-old lady with fibromyalgia attended a primary care clinic for the first time. She had just moved house and complained of severe neck and shoulder pain that had lasted for two weeks following the move, which was not settling. It turned out that she had been experiencing the symptoms for 15 years and she had recently attended a pain management programme and had just completed the final 12 month follow-up. She was tearful throughout the consultation and stated that she felt she may have damaged her neck in the move and her friends had told her that she should have a scan of her neck as she had probably done something serious to her spine. There were no abnormal findings when her doctor examined her. Firstly, the doctor listened and reassured her that she had not caused any serious damage in her neck from moving, she did not need a scan, and that she was probably experiencing an increase in her normal level of pain because her body was not accustomed to the physical activity involved in moving house. The doctor asked what Anusha had learnt on the pain management programme and if there was anything she could apply to help her in this situation. Anusha talked about pacing, exercises, and using thoughts and feelings. When asked if she was using these strategies, Anusha said she hadn't been using them for the last month, as she had been so busy with the move. The doctor encouraged her to start them up again. Anusha also mentioned that 'setbacks' had been mentioned on the programme, which are increases in pain that last for more than three days. The doctor urged her to try to use the setback plan from the programme and if she still had further problems to contact the pain management team. Anusha returned a month later to say that she had taken the doctor's advice, the setback had resolved and she was using her pain management strategies on a daily basis.

14.8 **Summary**

Long-term pain can be managed successfully in primary care. Trialling treatments early such as TENS, acupuncture and trigger-point injections against clearly stated functional outcomes and providing practical advice around staying active with pain can reduce the need for onward referral to a pain clinic. If in spite of these measures pain continues to cause considerable disability and suffering for the individual, referral to a pain clinic is recommended. Persistent pain is often best managed by a pain management programme; which have been shown to produce sustained benefits in this sometimes difficult group of patients.

Bibliography

Bath Pain Management Programme for Adolescents. www.bath.ac.uk/pain-management.

Burton, K. *et al. The Back Book* (2nd edn). Stationery Office Books, London.

Cochrane Collaboration; the reliable source of evidence in health care. www.cochrane.org.

Chapter 15

Working across boundaries in pain medicine

Trudy Towell

This chapter explores some of the issues which patients, their carers, GPs, hospital doctors, nurses and pain teams experience particularly when confronted with a challenging case. The findings of a critical study that examined the communication patterns between GPs and nurses providing palliative care in Australia highlighted difficulties patients' families face due to constant reassessments, the need to communicate information between different professionals and to update professionals on medication changes. The report identified that the patient often only received a few days' discharge medications, requiring the need to contact the GP. The GPs were often unaware that their patient was home and collaborative networking time was very limited for all professionals. Two case studies highlight the need for unambiguous decision making concerning patient management and interdisciplinary relationships.

15.1 Simon's acute abdominal pain

The first case study concerns Simon, 57-years-old and admitted to hospital with an acute abdomen. Unfortunately, at laparoscopy curative surgery was not possible due to widespread cancer. Postoperative pain relief was provided by an intravenous patient-controlled analgesia machine delivering morphine. Simon's pain was well controlled but he was nauseated requiring a combination of intravenous cyclizine and ondansetron. Simon's wife was very upset, but agreed to the involvement of the palliative care service who continued his opioids. However, Simon was experiencing unacceptable side-effects including nausea and excessive somnolence which he wanted to avoid so he could be alert and 'in control' for his last few weeks of life. Following multidisciplinary consultation including Simon and his wife, it was decided to insert a tunnelled epidural to provide analgesia, which could be continued at home.

Box 15.1 Communication requirements—tick when completed

- ❑ GP contacted and informed at least 24 hours prior to discharge
- ❑ Community nurses contacted prior to the patient's discharge. Training provided by the pain management team
- ❑ Pharmacist contact with the community pharmacist regarding the ongoing supply of the epidural or intrathecal pre-prepared syringes or bags
- ❑ Macmillan/palliative care nurse in hospital and community services/hospice contacted
- ❑ Risk assessment completed
- ❑ Patient/carer pack of information provided
- ❑ Equipment/alarms information
- ❑ Contact telephone numbers for the patient/carer to include GP, community nurse and pain management consultant
- ❑ Discharge letters: copied to the patient and faxed to the GP
- ❑ Pain management centre evaluation/communication sheet

Box 15.2 Patient/carers' preparation and education: instructions for equipment use and drug dosage/information

Tick when completed

- ❑ Setting up the device (where appropriate), e.g. programming and priming actions
- ❑ Alarm matrix and appropriate actions
- ❑ Changing the drug bags (or syringes)
- ❑ Monitoring the functioning of the device whilst in operation
- ❑ Monitoring of the insertion site
- ❑ Monitoring the effects and potential side-effects of the drugs being administered, including information and actions to be taken in the event of adverse drug reactions

The community nursing team visited Simon in hospital and training was provided by the nurse consultant and specialist nurses. Following discharge from hospital, this networking enabled cross-boundary partnerships with specialist nurses visiting the patient's home on a weekly basis, and visits by the patient to hospital to see the pain management consultant. It was pleasing to know that Simon was able to visit his local pub for a pint with his friends and attend a Sunday car boot sale with his wife.

Telephone follow-ups and a helpline for the pain team allowed communication between Simon, his wife, community nurses, his GP, the community pharmacist, specialist nurses and the pain management consultant. Simon died at home.

15.2 **Eileen's persistent abdominal pain**

The second case study involves Eileen, a 32-year-old with intermittent upper abdominal pain requiring frequent hospital admissions. Eileen had previously experienced pancreatitis following a cholecystectomy with sphincter of Oddi dysfunction. During each admission, junior ward doctors and ward nurses referred the patient to the pain team for advice and support as she always required rapidly increasing doses of morphine. Concurrently, Eileen and her husband demanded to see the pain team as she was distressed that the ward doctors and nurses were uncomfortable providing her with large and frequent doses of morphine.

On discharge from hospital, Eileen often requires oral morphine for several weeks, which is a concern to her GP and to her surgical consultant. Discharging patients from hospital on opioids can also be a concern of the pain team, especially if follow-up appointments are not arranged and patients do not have a stepwise weaning plan to discontinue morphine.

Complementary pain management therapies, e.g. transcutaneous electrical nerve stimulation (TENS), acupuncture and cognitive behavioural therapy, are often useful for these patients as well as injection therapies by the pain management consultant.

Figure 15.1 Crossing the boundaries. Utilizing the model below, this patient's ongoing management is supported by the visiting triangle (Figure 15.2)

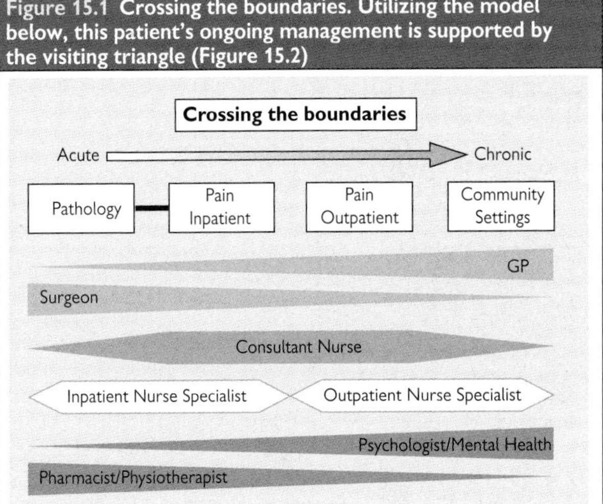

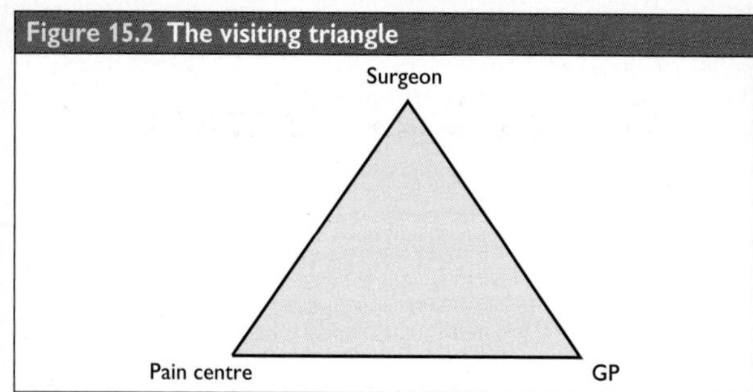

Figure 15.2 The visiting triangle

Each member of the team copies letters to each other and the pain team copies the letter to Eileen, which lists the agreed treatment plan and allows for Eileen's involvement, choice and compliance in her care. We hope this collaborative partnership will improve her long-term chronic pain management and reduce her admissions to hospital.

Both case studies demonstrate ways of interdisciplinary, cross-boundary working involving and maximizing the skills of a multiprofessional team.

Bibliography

Association for Palliative Medicine and The Pain Society (2005). The use of drugs beyond licence in palliative care and pain management. *APM and Pain Soc.* 1–10.

Mercadante, S. (1999). Review Article. Problems of long-term spinal opioid treatment in advance cancer patients. *Pain,* **79,** 1–3.

Pain Society (2003). Provisional recommendations for the appropriate use of opioids in patients with chronic non-cancer related pain. *Pain Soc.,* 1–20.

Queen's Medical Centre, Nottingham. Policy and Protocol for Discharging Patients with Infusion Devices in the Community Settings.

Street, A. and Blackford, J. (2001). Communication issues for the interdisciplinary community palliative care team. *J. Clin. Nurs.,* **10**(5), 643–650.

Chapter 16

Getting back to work

Cathy Price

There are some key questions to ask when having pain and thinking about going back to work. Why is work such a problem for people with pain, what is the right sort of help for people in pain, and when should this help be provided?

Managing long-term pain takes an enormous amount of resilience and fortitude. Not only must the person exercise and stretch every day, they must also plan and pace their activities. They may need to remember to take complex medication regularly and spend parts of the day using relaxation or distraction techniques to prevent flare-ups. In the workplace, where there are deadlines to be met and the schedule is often dictated by others and events around, managing pain can be a nightmare. Unsurprisingly, managing work is a major issue for people in continuous pain.

GPs have a crucial role to play as they are often the first port of call. They are aware that psychosocial factors and job satisfaction are important determinants. However, this knowledge does not seem to translate into practice; for example, in one study only a third of back pain sufferers were advised to stay active even though everyone working in this field acknowledges this to be true. There is confusion on what to say when someone is clearly struggling at work. Clear guidance on the right intervention at the right time is therefore needed. The following cases are based on actual cases and illustrate these dilemmas.

16.1 Michael's neck pain

Michael is a 47-year-old car production worker. He developed neck pain a few years ago which has increasingly become harder to manage. On the assembly line he needs to lift up and look up much of the day. He finds that he can manage but then he needs to take a lot of tablets to get through the day and by the time he gets home he just wants to lie down. He finds he is shouting at his wife and children. His supervisor can't see what all the fuss is about as he gets regular breaks like everyone else. Michael believes that his neck is wearing out because of the job and is asking for early retirement on medical grounds. As a primary care clinician, how would you respond?

16.2 Shirley's persistent pelvic pain

Shirley is 35-years-old with a history of treated endometriosis but has continuing pelvic pain. However, she found further management through a multidisciplinary pain clinic using amitriptyline, TENS and a brief pain management programme useful. She continues to do regular exercise. She also found the support given in helping her accept her pain invaluable. Shirley used to work as a secretary years ago and has no children, something she has also learned to accept through the local endometriosis support group. When she was in work she often phoned in sick with flare-up days. She is afraid that times have changed and she no longer has the skills to deal with modern office work. She would like to return to some sort of work and is asking your advice. Could you help her get back to work?

Before answering these questions, an overview of pain and work may help.

16.3 Size of the problem

Chronic pain, especially low back pain, is the leading health-related cause of time away from work and accounts for 28% of ill health benefit claims in the UK. Chronic pain is the UK's most costly health-care problem. Welfare payments stood at £3, 440 million in 1998 for back pain alone.

16.4 What are the health costs of unemployment?

Physical and mental morbidity associated with unemployment is high. Unemployed people are twice as likely to die within three years and three times as likely to commit suicide even after controlling for a wide variety of socioeconomic and health variables. After treatment in a multidisciplinary pain programme, workers were found to have better mental health and were more confident in managing their pain and general aspects of their lives than non-workers. It would seem that being in employment has positive health benefits in its own right. Getting there, however, is hard work. After one year's work absence, the chances of ever going back to work are very small indeed (Figure 16.1). Many chronic pain patients take a considerable time to accept that their pain is here to stay—often beyond a year. By that time the skills to manage work may have been lost.

Figure 16.1 Returning to work with pain (from Waddell, G. The *Back Pain Revolution*)

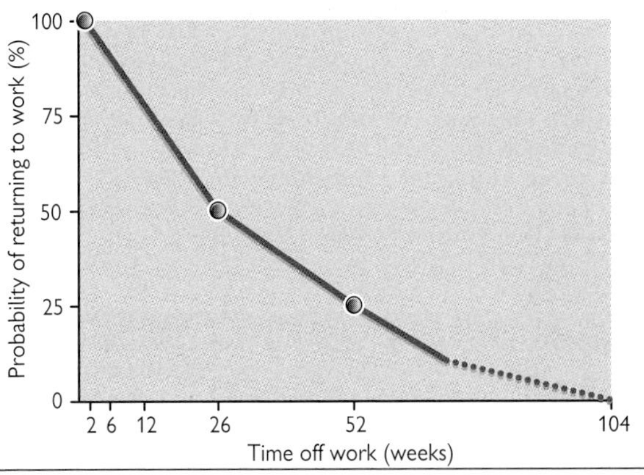

Box 16.1 Key factors predicting sick leave

- How likely someone thinks it is that they can go back to work
- Social support at work
- How harmful the pain seems
- Depression
- Pain intensity

(from Marhold, C., Linton S.J., and Melin, L. (2002) Identification of obstacles for chronic pain patients to return to work: evaluation of a questionnaire. *J. Occup. Rehab.* **12,** 65–75)

16.5 What are the key factors determining time away from work?

The frequency and duration of time away from work in those with pain depends more on individual and work-related psychosocial issues than the pain itself (Box 16.1). Common barriers for someone trying to stay in work or get back to work with long-term pain are:

- fear of re-injury
- difficulties with re-training
- poor recent employment history
- low confidence and self-esteem
- belief that benefits will be penalized

From the employer's perspective, possible barriers to hiring people with pain problems include difficulty in finding the right working conditions and fears of legal liability and discrimination. Many employers find, however, that a supportive environment can pay dividends. Despite all the help available, potential employees with chronic pain lack confidence and perceive unfavourable conditions which may not exist. Provision of care to bridge the gap between medical help and vocational rehabilitation schemes is badly needed.

A colour coded flag system has been developed to aid assessment of risk factors for continuing disability in chronic pain (Figure 16.2). Perhaps surprisingly, the pain itself plays little part. Use of the flags is a good way of systematically identifying barriers to work and could be done at an early stage by the GP.

Figure 16.2 Diagnostic triage for back pain

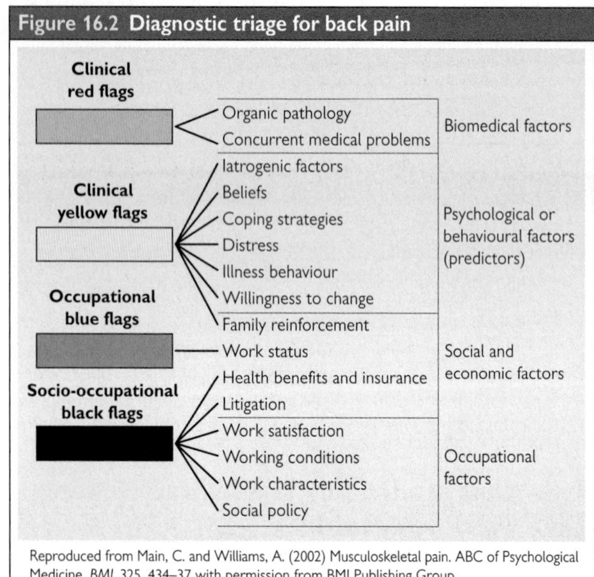

Reproduced from Main, C. and Williams, A. (2002) Musculoskeletal pain. ABC of Psychological Medicine. *BMJ*. 325, 434–37 with permission from BMJ Publishing Group.

16.6 General principles of treatment

Returning chronic pain patients to work is expensive and time-consuming. Success is more likely if sufferers are asked to tackle their beliefs about the cause of their pain rather than just focusing on treatments that tackle the pain itself. Most pain management programmes address general beliefs about pain. However, they do not tackle work-related beliefs and so do not return significant numbers to work. Programmes that confront specific work-related beliefs are more successful. Intervention plans are based on how long someone has been away from work.

16.7 Early intervention (0–4 weeks)

A positive attitude by the employer is important. Studies document reductions of up to 50% in both time lost from work and healthcare costs by taking action early on through telephoning, expressing concern, offering to take action and so on. *The Back Book* can be given to employees. This focuses on early resumption of activities and has been shown to reduce absence.

With the possible exception of spinal manipulation, clinical interventions are ineffective at an early stage. Lumbar belts and supports or traditional biomedical education as methods of preventing sickness do not work. There is insufficient evidence to advocate specific exercise or physical fitness programmes. The best early intervention is advice to stay active and this includes staying at work.

16.8 Intermediate intervention (4–8 weeks)

Managing this phase well is crucial. There is moderate evidence to support temporary work modification with the help of an advisor and focusing on rehabilitation, e.g. using pacing and the provision of a return to work package rather than single measures. The advisor should be skilled in dispute resolution and be able to provide incentives aimed at both the firm and the worker. This is cheaper than retraining in a new role. Occupational health practitioners can also offer advice by liaising with primary health care, the worker and the employer. **This is a crucial period and small focused interventions at this stage may be extremely effective.**

16.9 Late interventions

Once the person has gone beyond 12 weeks off work it is likely that they will require extensive rehabilitation and even alternative employment. The strength of belief of inability to return to work is highly predictive of failing to return to work after treatment. There is preliminary evidence that interventions which specifically address beliefs and attitudes may reduce future work loss. These interventions are characterized by a cognitive behavioural approach with self-management, reconditioning, vocational rehabilitation and psychological pain management (Box 16.2). Thus, overall there is a time progression to the level of intervention needed.

So how can we use this knowledge when looking at the case histories?

16.10 Back to Michael's neck pain

Michael needs a good explanation of pain along the lines of 'hurt doesn't mean harm', then the opportunity to try out movement in a graded fashion. Referral to a physiotherapist experienced in pain management is recommended. Michael is pushing himself hard at work, flaring up then resting, which will undo attempts at rehabilitation. Michael feels he has to do this to support his family. Paradoxically, he risks earning less money. Michael could try making some changes so that he takes frequent breaks and working half days for a short while. If Michael is having problems with his supervisor in a larger workplace, occupational health advisors can mediate on his behalf. In the first instance a letter from the treating healthcare professional or a phone call should be all that is needed.

As needed analgesia in the face of persistent poorly managed pain will lead to overdoing and reinforcement of activity patterns. Michael's GP should recommend regular analgesia and pacing. He could also point out the links between anger, frustration and increased pain. As the family doctor, he could help Michael to negotiate with his family for time out in the evening. Although these measures may seem time consuming, failure to act at this stage may lead to increased problems in the future with fixed patterns of behaviour, low self-esteem, high dependence on others and high consumption of medication.

Box 16.2 An active rehabilitation programme

- Education: directed at managing pain and overcoming disability
- Reassurance and advice to stay active
- Exercise: an active and progressive physical fitness programme
- Pain management: using behavioural principles
- Work: in an occupational setting and directed strongly towards return to work
- Rehabilitation: symptomatic relief measures should support and must not interfere with rehabilitation

16.11 **Back to Shirley's persistent pelvic pain**

Whilst Shirley has clearly made great strides in her pain management skills, she needs to gain confidence at work. She would benefit from a referral to a specific vocational rehabilitation programme. Here she would have the opportunity to problem solve with others, try out differing routines in a closely controlled environment, identify her personal skills and rehearse interviews. Knowledge of her rights as someone with a condition that is well known to cause disability would be helpful. A graded return to work programme using specific vocational schemes would be helpful once her beliefs about the potential harm of work are starting to shift. Thus whilst a GP would be unable to help Shirley directly, referral for specialist help is warranted.

Acknowledgement
With thanks to Dr Mark Saville, GP, for his helpful comments.

Figure 16.3 Returning to work

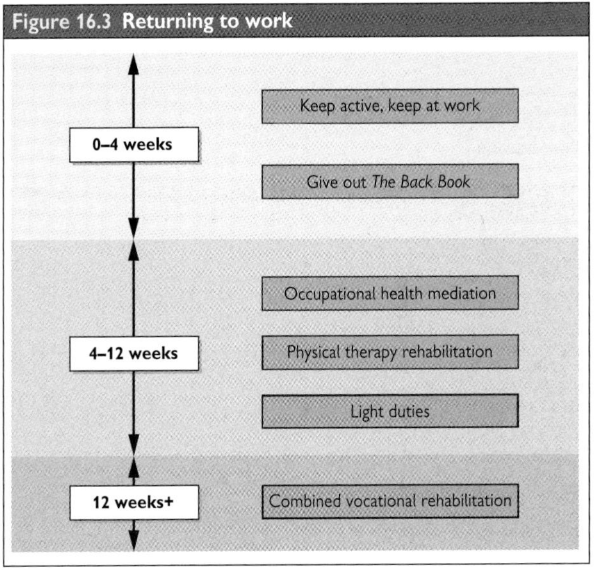

Bibliography

Burton, K. *et al. The Back Book* (2nd edn). Stationery Office Books, London.

Department for Work and Pensions (2002). Pathways to work: helping people into employment. HMSO, Norwich.

NHS Centre for Reviews and Dissemination (2000). Effective Health Care. Acute and Chronic Low Back Pain. **6**, 5.

Waddell G (1998). *The Back Pain Revolution*. Churchill Livingstone. London.

Index

O

P

R

S

T

U

V

W